THE LONGEVITY SOLUTION

Also by Kate Rowe-Ham:

Owning Your Menopause

THE LONGEVITY SOLUTION

21 days to health, strength & vitality

by Kate Rowe-Ham
founder of Owning Your Menopause

First published in Great Britain in 2026 by Yellow Kite
An imprint of Hodder & Stoughton Limited
An Hachette UK company

The authorised representative in the EEA is Hachette Ireland, 8 Castlecourt Centre, Dublin 15, D15 XTP3, Ireland (email: info@hbgi.ie)

1

Copyright © Kate Rowe-Ham 2026

The right of Kate Rowe-Ham to be identified as the Author of the Work has been asserted by her in accordance with the Copyright, Designs and Patents Act 1988.

Illustrations © WorkoutLabs, LLC, reproduced with their permission

All rights reserved. No part of this publication may be reproduced, stored in a retrieval system, or transmitted, in any form or by any means without the prior written permission of the publisher, nor be otherwise circulated in any form of binding or cover other than that in which it is published and without a similar condition being imposed on the subsequent purchaser.

A CIP catalogue record for this title is available from the British Library

The information in this book is not intended to replace or conflict with the advice given to you by your doctor or other health professional. All matters regarding your health should be discussed with your doctor. If you have any health concerns regarding the fitness plan, we recommend that you consult with your doctor before you embark on it. The author and publisher disclaim any liability directly or indirectly from the use of the material in this book by any person.

Trade Paperback ISBN 978 1 399 75155 1
ebook ISBN 978 1 399 75156 8

Typeset in Bembo MT by Hewer Text UK Ltd, Edinburgh
Printed and bound in Great Britain by Clays Ltd, Elcograf S.p.A.

Hodder & Stoughton policy is to use papers that are natural, renewable and recyclable products and made from wood grown in sustainable forests. The logging and manufacturing processes are expected to conform to the environmental regulations of the country of origin.

Hodder & Stoughton Limited
Carmelite House
50 Victoria Embankment
London EC4Y 0DZ

www.yellowkitebooks.co.uk

CONTENTS

Who Am I and Why Am I Writing This Book?   1
A Personal Insight   5
Why This Book Is Different   9

PART 1 THE SCIENCE OF LONGEVITY AND WHY IT MATTERS FOR WOMEN   13

Chapter 1	Epidemiology Meets the Blue Zones	17
Chapter 2	Healthspan vs Lifespan	27
Chapter 3	Women's Health Research and the Importance of Screening	31
Chapter 4	The Role of Female Hormones in Ageing	45
Chapter 5	Redefining Ageing	51
Chapter 6	Relationships and Their Impact on Health and Longevity	55

PART 2 THE THREE PILLARS OF LONGEVITY FOR WOMEN   63

PART 2.1 MOVEMENT   67

Chapter 7	Staying Strong and Independent	69
Chapter 8	Hormones, Ageing and Exercise	83

PART 2.2 NUTRITION   93

Chapter 9	Fuelling Your Body for Longevity	95

Chapter 10	Hormones, Ageing and Nutrition	105
Chapter 11	What to Eat to Support Your Mind and Slow Age-Related Cognitive Decline	109
Chapter 12	The Gut Feeling	113
Chapter 13	How to Eat: Mindful Eating and Intermittent Fasting	119
Chapter 14	Do Supplements Support?	125
Chapter 15	Unpacking UPFs: What's Really on Your Plate?	129
Chapter 16	Rethinking Alcohol's Role in a Long Life	133

PART 2.3 MENTAL WELL-BEING — 139

Chapter 17	Hormones, Ageing and Mental Resilience	143
Chapter 18	How Exercise Positively Influences the Mind for Longevity	149
Chapter 19	Connection and Purpose for Longevity	153
Chapter 20	Journalling	159
Chapter 21	Music for Motivation and Longevity	171
Chapter 22	Rest and Recovery: Slowing Down to Thrive	175
Chapter 23	Redefining Sleep for Longevity	179

PART 3 ASSESSING YOUR HEALTH — 183

| Chapter 24 | The Importance of Functional Fitness | 185 |
| Chapter 25 | So, Where Are You Right Now? | 189 |

PART 4 THE 21-DAY PLAN — 209

Chapter 26	Set Yourself up for Success	213
Chapter 27	Why the Exercises in This Plan Work for Longevity	217
Chapter 28	Journalling for the 21-Day Plan	225

Chapter 29	Alongside the Plan, Some Simple Exercise Hacks for Longevity	229
Chapter 30	Let's Go	233
Chapter 31	The Exercises	253

PART 5 MENUS, RECIPES AND MEAL PLANS — 291

What Does the Future Hold? — 317

Endnotes — 323
Index — 327
Acknowledgements — 337
About the Author — 339

You have a thousand problems in life until you have a health problem, and then you only have one.

Everything else, including money, relationships and stress, fades away in its shadow.

Suddenly, the things you once worried about seem so small because nothing else matters when your body or mind is screaming for help.

Health isn't just something you have, it's everything. It's the ability to wake up and feel alive, move freely, laugh without pain, and breathe without struggle. But we take it for granted, don't we? Until it's gone, we don't truly understand how precious it is. When your health is compromised every little thing becomes harder. Dreams get put on hold. Happiness feels distant, and life's colours start to fade.

That's why taking care of yourself isn't a luxury. It's an act of love, a gift to your future self.

Because when you're healthy, you can face anything. Without it, even the smallest battles feel impossible.

Don't wait to lose it to realise its value.

WHO AM I AND WHY AM I WRITING THIS BOOK?

I'm Kate Rowe-Ham, a women's fitness coach, entrepreneur, author of *Owning Your Menopause: Fitter, Calmer, Stronger in 30 Days* and founder of the Owning Your Menopause Fitness App. Through my work and the thriving community I've built, I've witnessed women's incredible potential to thrive during midlife and beyond when armed with the right tools, knowledge and habits.

However, this book is about more than menopause. It's about extending your years and enhancing the quality of those years. Longevity is not simply about living longer; it's about living better, ensuring your life is vibrant, independent and fulfilling, regardless of age. In a world where quick fixes and trendy fads dominate health, I want to offer something different: a guide grounded in science, sustainability and practical action.

At the heart of this book is a 21-day habit-setting transformation suitable for any stage of life. Whether you're just beginning to consider improving your long-term health or you've already started making changes, this programme has been designed to meet you where you are. It's a simple yet powerful framework for building habits that support vitality, independence and joy – not just for now, but for life.

And here's something I strongly encourage: don't do this alone. Longevity isn't just an individual pursuit; it's something we can and should strive for together. I would love you to invite your parents or other loved ones to join you in this journey, because the habits and insights you'll gain from the tests and activities in the book can open your eyes to how small, intentional changes can drastically improve your quality of life and theirs. I got my mum and her partner to test them all out for you and it has been amazing to see their progress.

Creating positive change is only the beginning. The key to longevity isn't just about making changes but sustaining them for life. Too often, we implement healthy habits, see improvements, and slowly drift back into old patterns. It's human nature and one of the most significant barriers I see to long-term success.

This book is as much about maintaining habits as it is about forming them. The changes we'll explore together aren't temporary fixes; they're meant to become a part of who you are. They're habits that support your health today and your vitality for years to come. My goal is to provide you with the tools, strategies and mindset shifts necessary to maintain these habits for life.

When I talk about longevity in the book, I reference the Blue Zones, where people are not only living longer, but thriving well into later life. In these communities, people move naturally throughout their day, eat mostly whole, plant-based foods, maintain strong social connections, find meaning and purpose, and live in ways that help reduce stress and protect their health over the long term.

But here's something important: you don't need to live in Sardinia, Okinawa or Nicoya to experience the benefits of a Blue Zone lifestyle. You can create your own version of a Blue Zone, right at home. Your kitchen, your dining table, your routines, even the way you connect with others, all of these can become foundations for a longer, stronger and more fulfilling life.

That's what I would like you to think about when you read this book and do the plan. It's about taking the science and wisdom of longevity and making it accessible, practical and sustainable for you wherever you live. My passion for this work comes from watching how powerful even the smallest changes can be, not just in my own life but in the lives of the women and families I work with. I've seen how introducing movement, improving the food we eat and building stronger connections can completely transform the way people feel about their health and their future.

I hope that as you continue through these pages, you'll feel inspired to shape your own environment in ways that support you to make your home a place that doesn't just keep you alive but helps you truly thrive. And when you do that, you're not just improving your own health; you're creating ripples of change that can positively influence your family, your friends, and even your wider community.

A PERSONAL INSIGHT

As I write this, my mum is 77 years old. She's vibrant, active and has a wonderful sense of community. That social connection has always been important to her. Still, in recent years, I've come to understand just how vital it is not only for emotional well-being but also for longevity itself. She is also my only remaining parent, living abroad, so I have dug deep into this research to see how I can help her live a better, more enjoyable life, pain-free and hopefully disease-free.

Her life has not been without challenges. She's faced cancer and undergone radiotherapy, a journey that has understandably left its mark both physically and emotionally. Alongside that, she has lived with food phobias and a thought, like most of us, that smaller is better. These fears shaped her relationship with eating in ways that are far more common than many people realise, especially among women of her generation. Her story is one I see reflected again and again in the women I work with, women who never truly learned how to eat for health and vitality, only how to restrict or react.

The more I learn about ageing and longevity, the more I see how the three pillars of movement, nutrition, and mental well-being are not just important; they are inseparable. They shape not only how long we live but also how we feel in our bodies, how we cope with life's inevitable stressors and how empowered we are to keep showing up for ourselves.

My mum has always been active, but until recently, she'd never paid attention to building bone or muscle strength. Like many women, she thought walking and staying busy would be enough. However, as we age, resistance training becomes essential not only to prevent falls or frailty but also to preserve independence and confidence. With gentle encouragement, she began incorporating light-strength exercises into her routine. The transformation was subtle at first: an easier time getting up from a chair, fewer complaints about aches but, over time, something far more powerful emerged: belief in her own capability. She now feels stronger, more stable and more optimistic about the years ahead.

But movement alone isn't the full picture. Longevity also lives in our kitchens – in our habits around food and nourishment. For my mum, food has long been associated with worry. Her past health experiences left her cautious and uncertain. She wasn't eating badly, but she wasn't eating with confidence or joy either. Helping her rebuild a sense of trust in food has been one of the most meaningful parts of this journey. We didn't overhaul everything overnight; instead, we made small, manageable changes, adding protein-rich snacks, focusing on fibre and trying colourful, wholefood meals that felt safe and doable. Bit by bit, she began to notice the difference, not just in her energy, but also in her mindset. She felt more fuelled, more stable, more herself.

And then, perhaps most importantly, there's mental well-being. My mum is incredibly lucky in this area. She has a close-knit group of friends who surround her with warmth, laughter and a sense of purpose. I see the impact that connection has on her every single day. She's not isolated; she's engaged. Her conversations are meaningful, her outings frequent. That community has held her through cancer, through grief, through fear. It is, without exaggeration, one of the most powerful contributors to her longevity.

We often underestimate the power of purpose, of feeling seen and valued. However, the evidence is clear: those who feel connected – whether through friendships, family or community – not only live longer but also live better. They navigate challenges with more resilience, and they face ageing with more grace.

My mum's story is not about perfection. It's about what's possible, how even in our seventies, even after illness, even with fear in the background, we can start layering in new habits that support a longer, stronger life. Her journey reminds me that strength takes many forms and that the path to longevity begins with compassion, curiosity and a willingness to try.

WHY THIS BOOK IS DIFFERENT

I want this book to highlight the disparities between men and women because, for too long, longevity research and advice has been centred on men, even though women, on average, live six to eight years longer than men. Historically, women were excluded from clinical trials due to hormonal complexity, and much of women's health research has focused narrowly on reproduction, neglecting the broader physical and mental shifts that occur across the lifespan. While women may live longer due to biological advantages like oestrogen's protective effects and genetic resilience, they often experience an extended period of poor health in later years, with up to 50% of women over 50 suffering from osteoporosis and nearly two-thirds of Alzheimer's patients being female.[1] This book aims to challenge and change the conversation, empowering you to take control of your long-term health and vitality through a targeted approach built on three essential pillars: movement, nutrition and mental well-being.

Unlike other longevity books that focus on biohacking, expensive supplements or complex medical interventions, *The Longevity Solution* is grounded in simple, sustainable habits that have a profound impact.

Before you start the 21-Day Plan, Part 1 will discuss the science behind longevity and why it matters, particularly for women. Part 2 focuses on the three pillars of longevity for women: more movement, improved nutrition and good mental well-being.

Part 3 begins by guiding you through key health assessments: powerful predictors of long-term health that help identify risk factors early, allowing you to take proactive steps to offset age-related diseases such as heart disease, osteoporosis and cognitive decline. Part 4 introduces the 21-Day Plan, which shows how by following structured, daily actions that fit seamlessly into your lifestyle, you will build a framework to protect against frailty, nourish your body to maintain optimal energy, and develop a resilient mindset to handle life's transitions with strength and confidence.

When you get to the workout section, you will have access to a unique QR code that will take you to videos that bring each session to life in real time. I'll be right there with you, guiding you through. And if you'd rather work from the book, everything you need is here in these pages. Alongside the exercises are the meal plans, ensuring you are nourishing your body – these are not intended for weight loss but to show you how you need to eat well alongside exercise.

While average lifespans have increased, the number of years we spend in good health – our healthspan – has not. More people are reaching old age, but often with years of illness, reduced independence and poor quality of life. The good news is that longevity isn't just determined by luck or genetics. Research shows that only 10–20% of how long we live comes from our DNA.[2] Daily choices shape the rest: how we move, what we eat, how we manage stress, sleep and connection. You have far more control over how you age than you might think. Every small habit you build today helps create a future filled with energy, strength and joy.

The Longevity Solution will help you future-proof your body and mind, ensuring that you not only add years to your life but also add life to your years.

I love that sentence. Reread it. Longevity isn't just about adding years to your life; it's about adding life to your years. It's not simply about avoiding death; it's about truly learning how to live. To live a long life, you must wake up each day with energy, feel strong and capable in your body, and stay active and engaged in the things that bring you joy.

For me, longevity means being able to run around with my kids (or grandkids) pain-free, without feeling out of breath, and knowing that my body will support me in doing the things I love, not hold me back. It's about keeping my mind sharp, my bones strong and my heart full.

PART 1
The Science of Longevity and Why It Matters for Women

I'm deeply passionate about helping women live fuller, healthier and more vibrant lives because far too many of us are running on empty. In the UK today, women are being stretched more than ever before. We're the caregivers, professionals, partners and emotional anchors in our families and communities. We hold so much together, but too often our own needs quietly fall to the bottom of the list.

It's time that changed.

As I have mentioned, true longevity is about quality years, not quantity. It's about having the energy, strength and confidence to enjoy life on our terms, to feel independent for as long as we can, and that means taking ownership of our health now, not someday. Because let's be honest: life never really slows down. The demands just shift and grow, and we will never find the right time.

From working with thousands of women, I know that midlife can feel like a pressure cooker. We're navigating physical changes, hormonal shifts, muscle loss, disrupted sleep and increased health risks, all while managing careers, family responsibilities, ageing parents and often teenage or grown children. Add to that the emotional load we carry, and it's no wonder we feel overwhelmed, anxious or burned out.

Yet, despite everything we do for others, we rarely give ourselves permission to pause and prioritise what we need. Exercise and nutrition often feel like yet another thing on an endless to-do list. We delay it until the kids are older, until work calms down, until we feel more motivated. But that perfect time never arrives. Meanwhile, our bodies and minds are crying out for attention. Then there's the hidden element that many of us don't realise: the more we delay, the more we impact our future health.

That's why I created this book and the 21-Day Plan. I want to help you build habits that fit into your life, engage in exercises focused on strengthening your mind and body and introduce moments of calm through journalling, rather than adding to your stress. It's not about radical overhauls or impossible routines. It's about real, sustainable changes that meet you where you are. We'll focus on three powerful pillars: movement, nutrition and mental well-being. These are the foundations of long-term health, and they are more accessible than you might think, with the right mindset and support.

Movement doesn't have to involve punishing workouts or hours spent in the gym. It can be joyful, empowering and profoundly transformative, especially when it helps manage menopause symptoms, strengthens bones and muscles and enhances mental clarity. Similarly, nourishing your body doesn't mean adhering to strict diets; it's about fuelling yourself with food that supports energy, brain health and resilience. As for your mental well-being, it's not a luxury; it's the glue that holds everything together. Learning to manage stress, improve sleep and set boundaries is essential not just for you but for everyone who relies on you.

Because here's the thing: we can't pour from an empty cup. And while many of us have mastered the art of pushing through, true strength comes from knowing when to stop, reset and choose ourselves.

We're not too late. We're not too old. We're not too busy. We just need a roadmap and someone who understands what this chapter of life feels like.

I also passionately believe in the ripple effect. When we commit to taking care of ourselves, we set a powerful example for the next generation. We show our daughters, nieces and younger peers that self-care is not selfish – it's necessary. It's smart. It's strong. We teach them that they don't have to wait for burnout, illness or crisis to prioritise their well-being.

So, let this be your starting point. Use the next 21 days as an opportunity to reset, not with guilt or pressure, but with purpose and clarity. This is about making changes that will serve you for years to come. I'll be right here with you every step of the way.

Because you deserve to live the years ahead with joy, energy and freedom, and the time to start isn't someday. It's today.

CHAPTER 1

Epidemiology Meets the Blue Zones

Epidemiology studies how diseases spread, who is affected by them, and why. It helps us determine what causes illnesses and how to prevent them. Epidemiologists investigate these questions. They study disease patterns, ageing and lifestyle choices in different populations to learn how to live longer, healthier lives.

Observing health patterns involves tracking the prevalence of diseases, identifying where they are most common, and determining who is most affected. This helps identify trends, such as whether a disease increases or decreases over time or if certain populations are more vulnerable. Comparing groups involves examining individuals with a disease and those without it to identify potential causes or risk factors. The focus on groups of people and populations is central. Unlike clinical medicine, which focuses on individuals, epidemiology views the community as the patient. For example, suppose one group of women has a high rate of heart disease, perhaps in this case women who are post-menopause. In that case, epidemiologists investigate lifestyle habits, medical history and environmental exposures that might explain the reason. Using these methods, epidemiologists can understand how diseases develop, identify who is most at risk and develop effective strategies for prevention and treatment.

Epidemiology does not just help us understand health in faraway places. It also shows us what's happening in our communities. For example, in the UK, women have an average life expectancy of 83 years. However, living without serious health problems means their healthy life expectancy is only 63 years.[3] This suggests that many women spend the last 20 years of their lives dealing with chronic illnesses, a reality that doesn't align with the vision of a vibrant and fulfilling later life.

Then there's the reality of the postcode lottery in life expectancy. Women in deprived areas live 7 years less than those in wealthier neighbourhoods.[4] This difference isn't just about individual choices, it highlights broader societal issues, such as access to fresh food, safe green spaces, lower stress levels and good healthcare. The idea that our environment can influence our longevity reminds us of the importance of public health policy and social conditions.

While 75.7% of women in the UK report feeling healthy, half (50.1%) live with at least one long-term health condition, and 22.3% indicate that health problems limit their daily activities.[5] These issues aren't always directly linked to ageing, of course, many stem from chronic stress, lifestyle factors or inequality. The most common conditions include joint pain and arthritis, anxiety and depression, cardiovascular disease, asthma, type 2 diabetes, gut issues like IBS, migraines and pelvic health concerns such as incontinence. Dementia and Alzheimer's disease account for 12.7% of female deaths,[6] making them the leading causes of death among women. Meanwhile, breast cancer remains a major health threat, particularly in women aged 50 to 64.

And the truth is that many women haven't had the support, education or space to make lasting changes that could help prevent or alleviate these challenges. That's precisely why conversations like this matter, because you can change. It's never too late to take back control of your health.

Epidemiology isn't just about studying problems but also about finding solutions. We already know that regular physical activity, a balanced diet and good mental health are key to longevity and can significantly improve health outcomes. The challenge is making these habits accessible and sustainable for everyone, not just those with the time, money and knowledge to prioritise their health.

The Blue Zones

Now that we've dipped our toes into epidemiology and how it helps us uncover the stories that health statistics tell us, I want to explain how I became a little obsessed with longevity and wanted to learn more about it. Let's take a little trip around the globe to discover where people are quietly, happily and impressively outliving the rest of us.

My interest began with a Netflix documentary called *Live to 100: Secrets of the Blue Zones,* which explores the connection between epidemiology and longevity, rooted in the concept of Blue Zones. Dan Buettner, a National Geographic explorer and journalist, dedicated years to researching the longest-living populations and brought this idea to life. He believes it's not about preventing death but about learning to live. He wanted to discover if it was possible to reverse the process of ageing. Dan has invested over 20 years trying to achieve that. Rather than seeking answers in petri dishes or test tubes, he identified five places worldwide where people achieve remarkable longevity.

Some locations are islands, others are mountainous, some are incredibly remote and some are surprisingly urban. While varying on the surface, they all adhere to the same formula that produces the longest-lived individuals on the planet.

These are the communities that make epidemiologists do a double-take. Not because people there are doing anything particularly flashy, but precisely because they aren't. There are no extreme workouts, obsessive calorie counting or 17-step wellness morning routines. Yet they're living longer, stronger and with fewer chronic health conditions than many of us are navigating in midlife and beyond.

As someone who works with women, encouraging them to make fundamental lifestyle changes every day, I love the Blue Zones. They resemble a real-life Pinterest board in terms of longevity. The best part is that they encompass everything I discuss in this book and my previous one. The habits are simple, sustainable and transferable. You don't have to uproot your life and move to Okinawa (though if you do, please send a postcard).

However, here's the critical point: we might never have identified these regions without the use of epidemiology. Sardinia's rugged hill towns and Ikaria's sleepy olive groves would have remained beautiful places to visit. It's epidemiologists who spotted the trends: people here weren't just living longer; they were living better with energy, independence and connection into their nineties and beyond.

The Blue Zones, in turn, provided epidemiology with something it rarely receives: tangible evidence. And here's the thing: these communities aren't health-obsessed. They engage in natural movement, primarily consume plants, maintain social connections and live purposefully.

I spoke recently with a woman in my community who said, 'I want to be the 90-year-old who can still carry her shopping, not someone waiting for help.' That's the Blue Zone spirit. And it's what good epidemiological data offers us: a list of risks and a vision of what's possible.

Therefore, it is essential to understand epidemiology and the Blue Zones in tandem. It's not a one-way street; it's a proper friendship. Blue Zones provide us with a lifestyle blueprint, and epidemiology backs it up with evidence, helping us understand why these habits are effective and how we can incorporate them into our own lives, regardless of our location.

The most powerful takeaway for me is that these are ordinary people. They're not biohacking or chasing youth but are ageing with grace, strength and joy. And the real secret of the Blue Zones isn't where they are on the map; it's what they do every day. And we can start building that into our own lives, one walk, one wholesome meal, one good laugh at a time.

Where are the Blue Zones?

The story begins with two researchers – Dr Gianni Pes and Dr Michel Poulain – who studied areas with unusually high concentrations of centenarians. While mapping a cluster of long-lived individuals in Sardinia, Italy, they used a blue pen to circle the region with the highest concentration of individuals. This circled area became known as the first Blue Zone.

This early discovery caught the attention of author and explorer Dan Buettner, who partnered with National Geographic and a team of demographers, scientists and medical researchers to dig deeper. Together, they set out to identify additional regions around the world that shared this remarkable trend of longevity.

The five areas around the globe that they discovered, known as Blue Zones, house some of the longest-living and healthiest people on Earth. While the locations differ greatly, the common thread is straightforward: movement, connection, purpose and nourishment from whole foods. These communities don't pursue longevity; it's ingrained in their daily habits. Here's an overview of each zone and the lessons we can learn from them:

Sardinia, Italy

Rugged hills, stone paths and a life lived outdoors. Women are the matriarchs of multi-generational homes, deeply respected and central to daily life. Sardinian women tend to remain active into old age, engaging in activities such as gardening, cooking, walking and lifting grandchildren, and often outlive the men. Their routines are carefully woven with purpose. They nourish others, manage family life and maintain strong female friendships, all while following the same Mediterranean diet. Age brings wisdom, not invisibility, and their role grows stronger with time. Family comes first, stress is low and ageing is embraced, not feared.

Okinawa, Japan

In Okinawa, life is shaped by gardens, laughter and a deep sense of purpose. Okinawan women hold the record for the longest lifespans in the world, a fact largely attributed to their traditional diet, which is rich in sweet potatoes, tofu, seaweed and turmeric. They follow the practice of *hara hachi bu* – eating until they are about 80% full, which helps maintain a healthy weight and avoid overeating. Lifelong friendships are nurtured within tight-knit social groups called *moai*, which offer emotional support and a strong sense of belonging.

Central to Okinawan life is the concept of *ikigai*, a Japanese term that means 'reason for being'. Rooted in the words *iki* (life) and *gai* (worth or value), ikigai represents the joy found in living a purposeful life. It's this sense of meaning that keeps many Okinawans active, resilient and fulfilled well into old age. The research indicates that having a clear purpose not only enhances mental well-being but also promotes longevity and strengthens the body's ability to cope with stress and disease. It is one of the most powerful longevity tools and I truly believe that this is the way to add good years to your life.

Ikaria, Greece

Life on the island of Ikaria moves to a different rhythm, one defined by steep, winding paths, unhurried mornings and a diet rooted in the gifts of the land. Meals are rich in wild greens, beans, olive oil and herbal teas, all sourced locally and prepared with care. Ikarians embrace daily naps, dance late into the night at lively village festivals and share laughter and stories with their neighbours. Chronic diseases such as heart disease and diabetes are rare; dementia is almost unheard of. Here, time feels fluid, unbound by the pressures of the outside world. Deep social connections, simple pleasures and a strong sense of community weave through everyday life, forming the foundation for the Ikarians' remarkable health and longevity.

Nicoya Peninsula, Costa Rica

In Nicoya, life is anchored by early mornings, the shade of mango trees and a deep sense of community. At the heart of their remarkable longevity is the *plan de vida*, a strong, guiding sense of purpose that keeps Nicoyans active, engaged and optimistic well into their nineties and beyond. Daily life is grounded in physical activity, often woven naturally into farming, walking and tending to family duties. Meals are simple yet nourishing: plates filled with black beans, rice, corn tortillas and an abundance of fresh tropical fruits. Their water, rich in calcium and magnesium, supports strong bones and vibrant health. Mealtimes are never rushed; they are about gathering with family, sharing conversation and reinforcing the bonds that sustain both body and spirit.

Loma Linda, California

In the heart of Southern California, Loma Linda stands out as a rare pocket of longevity in the United States. Much of this can be credited to the lifestyle of its large community of Seventh-Day Adventists, whose habits promote long, healthy lives. Many Adventists follow a predominantly plant-based diet, centred on legumes, whole grains, vegetables and nuts, while intentionally avoiding alcohol, caffeine and processed foods. The Sabbath, observed from Friday evening to Saturday evening, is considered a sacred day dedicated to rest, spiritual reflection, time in nature and reconnecting with family and friends. Movement is naturally incorporated into their routines through activities such as walking and gardening, and they stay physically engaged well into old age. In Loma Linda, community bonds are strong, faith is a guiding force, and a commitment to both physical and spiritual well-being shapes each day.

> You don't need to live in a Blue Zone to thrive.
>
> You can create your own right here, right now.
>
> One habit, one choice, one day at a time.

This is your longevity solution.

Longevity isn't just about good genes or sheer luck; it's about our daily habits, environment and choices. You don't have to live in a Blue Zone to improve longevity. Each of us can start where we are, with what we have, and take small, meaningful steps every day, which is where the 21-Day Plan comes into play. We should consider longevity now, long before problems arise. And if it all feels overwhelming, just remember that epidemiologists have already conducted the research, and I have made it accessible here.

Now, all you need to do is follow the 21-Day Plan, stick to it, and incorporate the lessons from this book into your daily life for ever. And when you begin your plan, please remember that what distinguishes these places is not a singular secret but a mix of daily habits, diets, social norms and mindsets that support vibrant, healthy ageing.

CHAPTER 2

Healthspan vs Lifespan

A few months ago, a client came to me. At 46, she had just received a diagnosis of osteopenia. She expressed her disbelief, saying she thought it was something that only happened to people in their seventies, half-laughing and half-panic-stricken. She had always viewed herself as relatively healthy: she walked her dog daily and ate well, but strength training had never been part of her routine. It always seemed like something for other people: younger individuals, gym enthusiasts and those with more time. Not her.

But this diagnosis shook her. It wasn't just about her bones; it was a wake-up call. For the first time, she began to think about her future differently. Not only about how long she might live, but also about how well she wanted to live as she aged. That's when the conversation turned to something most of us don't talk about nearly enough: the difference between lifespan and healthspan.

Lifespan is exactly what it sounds like: the number of years you live. That number appears on the birthday card or, eventually, on your death certificate. However, healthspan is far more significant in the day-to-day reality of life. It's the number of years you stay well, mobile, strong, independent, mentally sharp and enjoying the things you love. You might live to 92, but if the last 20 years are spent managing multiple health conditions, struggling to move without pain or relying on others to get through the day, that's a long period of surviving, not thriving. On the other hand, someone might live to 82 and remain active, energised and autonomous until their final weeks. That's healthspan.

My client told me, 'I want to be the mum who still hikes with her kids when they're in their twenties. I want to carry my suitcase and run up the stairs when I'm in my sixties and seventies.' And that's when we started. Nothing dramatic. Ten minutes a day of simple resistance training, using her body weight, bands and light weights. No fancy gym, no complicated programme, just consistent, focused movement to build strength and stability.

Over time, things began to shift. Her posture improved. Her confidence grew. She felt more solid in her body, less achy, more in control. Her following bone scan showed no further loss, but even more importantly, she felt better in her skin. 'I don't feel like I'm waiting for things to worsen anymore,' she told me. 'I feel like I'm building something.'

I want every woman to understand this: midlife isn't a decline; it's a transition. And it's the perfect time to start supporting your future self. You don't need to overhaul your life overnight, but what you do now matters more than ever. I will discuss this further in the next chapter, but after the age of 40, we naturally experience a decline in muscle mass, bone density and metabolic resilience. Hormonal shifts can amplify that process, making it harder to feel strong and energised. But it's also the moment we can impact our trajectory the most. The sooner we invest in our healthspan, the longer we'll enjoy the years ahead.

Think of healthspan as your years of good living. The truth is, no one wants to just live longer if it means being trapped in a body that doesn't work. We want to dance in the kitchen at 70. We want to travel at 75 without worrying about our balance. We want to lift our grandkids, carry our shopping, garden, swim, laugh and move with freedom. We want to feel alive for as many years as possible, not just in the present.

So, if you've noticed some shifts, please understand it's not too late.

Think of it like this: if lifespan is the length of this book, healthspan is the quality of the story inside. So, let's do our best to ensure it's a brilliant one.

CHAPTER 3

Women's Health Research and the Importance of Screening

Let's get one thing straight from the start – understanding what's going on with our minds, bodies and relationships as we age isn't just nice to know . . . it's vital. Because once you know what's happening, you can do something about it. And honestly, when you hit midlife, there's often a lot happening all at once, isn't there?

There are the hormonal shifts, of course, that fun roller-coaster of mood changes, hot flushes, sleep drama and wondering if you're losing your mind because you can't remember the name of that thing you just saw on the thing . . . you know what I mean. Then there's the change in roles. Maybe your kids don't need you quite as much, or your parents need you more. Careers shift. Relationships evolve. You can start to feel a little invisible. A little lost. We will cover this later, but here's the thing: this can also be the most powerful time in your life.

When we stop and take stock, we realise that now is the time to future-proof ourselves. We don't need fads or quick fixes; we need small, sustainable habits that actually work for us. And we need to talk about women's health in a way that finally makes sense.

So, let me be clear: women's health is about so much more than periods, pregnancy and menopause. It's heart disease. It's dementia. It's bone health, gut health, mood, energy and muscle. Fertility, pregnancy and menopause are essential, but they are only part of the picture. Women age differently, metabolise medication differently, and face greater risks for conditions like osteoporosis and dementia.[7]

Here's the maddening bit, though: for years, women were simply left out of the conversation. Literally. Did you know women weren't properly included in clinical trials until the 1990s? I was shocked when I found that out. Back in 1977, the US Food and Drug Administration (FDA) told researchers to exclude any woman who might become pregnant from early-stage studies. They didn't want to risk harming a potential foetus, but the result? Entire generations of women were left without proper medical data. Treatments were tested mostly on men, with male bodies as the norm, and we've been paying the price ever since.[8]

Think about it: the leading cause of death for women is heart disease.[9] Yet for years, it was researched almost entirely in men. Most people associate heart attacks with dramatic chest pain. Yet for women, symptoms are often subtler, including nausea, jaw pain and fatigue, and women are seven times more likely than men to be misdiagnosed during a heart attack. Even the way drugs were dosed didn't account for our biology. Our hormones were seen as an inconvenience, so male bodies got all the attention. Can you believe that?

Things have improved since then. In 1993, the National Institutes of Health (NIH) made it mandatory to include women in US federally funded research, and the UK eventually followed suit. But that early damage created a knowledge gap we're still trying to close. Even now, women, especially women of colour, are underrepresented in research, and it shows in our care.[10]

And let's talk about hormone replacement therapy for a sec. Remember the panic around HRT in the early 2000s? When the Women's Health Initiative study linked HRT to breast cancer and heart issues, women ran for the hills. But what hardly anyone said out loud was that the average age of the women in the study was 63. Well past menopause. Later research found that starting HRT earlier, closer to the onset of menopause, comes with very different risks and, in many cases, a lot of benefits. But by then, so much fear had set in. And so many women were left to suffer in silence.

It makes me angry to think of how many of us just got on with it, considering we had no other option. That confusion around HRT isn't just poor communication, and it's a symptom of a much bigger problem: when women aren't properly researched, our care falls short. We deserve better.

We are moving in the right direction. HRT is now safer, doses are lower, and it's far more personalised.[11] But it's still not a magic wand, and it's not for everyone. What is for everyone is the right to informed, compassionate, personalised care. You should feel empowered, not overwhelmed by your choices.

But even now, the inequality continues. Did you know that in 2019, the *Guardian* reported that female-specific conditions like endometriosis receive less research funding than erectile dysfunction? We still know this is true today. That's not just frustrating, it's enraging. We've still got a long way to go, but women's voices are getting louder. Organisations are finally starting to listen. And people like you, reading this book, are a big part of that shift.

So, if you've ever felt unheard, dismissed or like you've had to figure things out alone, you're not imagining it. But you're not alone anymore. This book is here to help you make sense of what's going on, give you the tools you need to feel strong and informed and, most importantly, remind you that it's never too late to take your health into your own hands.

This isn't about chasing youth or unrealistic ideals. It's about feeling good, being strong, staying independent and showing up for yourself in a way that feels aligned, doable and yours.

Why This Matters

The exclusion of women from medical research has real, ongoing consequences. Treatments may not be optimised for women's bodies. Symptoms of life-threatening conditions can be misdiagnosed or missed altogether.

Osteoporosis is one example. Women are at much higher risk, yet bone health isn't prioritised until fractures occur. Prevention strategies should start far earlier.

Dementia also disproportionately affects women, but links between menopause, hormones and brain health remain under-researched.[12] Brain health and menopause should be discussed together, but they are rarely addressed.

And if there's one glaring area where the gender health gap persists, it's menopause. Every woman will experience it, yet for decades, it has been poorly understood, underresearched and often dismissed. Symptoms like brain fog, anxiety, exhaustion and joint pain have been minimised, leaving many women to just get on with it without adequate support.

Thankfully, the conversation is changing. Awareness is growing, and more women are demanding better education, more equitable workplace policies and increased access to treatment. Still, we have work to do.

We need more research that treats women as biologically distinct, not smaller versions of men. We need better diagnosis and care for female-specific conditions. We need to invest more in education about menopause and midlife health. We must address the inequalities that mean where you live and your income level can determine your health outcomes.

Women's health isn't a niche; it's the health of half the population.[13]

- If something feels wrong, push for answers.
- If a doctor dismisses you, seek a second opinion.
- If menopause is affecting your life, find the proper support and treatment.
- If healthcare policies neglect women's health, speak up and demand change.

Your health matters, today, tomorrow and for the long, vibrant life you deserve.

Screening for Women and Why It Matters for Longevity

I'll admit it – I've been guilty of putting things off. Between juggling work, family and the general busyness of life, it's all too easy to brush aside a screening letter or think, I feel fine, I don't need this right now. But here's the uncomfortable truth: the moments when we delay these health checks can be the very moments that dictate our future. Regarding longevity, prevention is not just better than a cure, it's everything.

After my dad died in 2022 at the age of 75 from cancer, I began to question some of my abnormal symptoms. I have always been susceptible to bloating and my gut often fluctuated between constipation and diarrhoea; not all the time but often enough to notice. I later discovered that my granny had bowel cancer in her sixties. My sister was diagnosed in her late thirties with Crohn's disease, so I saw this as an opportunity to advocate for some investigations. Had my dad reacted earlier to some of his symptoms, he might have had a better chance of living longer. As it turns out, I have SPS – Serrated Polyposis Syndrome – something I had never even heard of before. Like many, I assumed colon cancer was a risk for older men or those with symptoms, but SPS is different. It causes multiple serrated polyps in the colon, some of which have a high risk of becoming cancerous. It was only through advocating for my health that these polyps were discovered, making me realise how crucial early detection is. Many people with SPS remain undiagnosed as it often presents no warning signs. Risk factors include family history, genetic predisposition and age, with most diagnoses occurring after age 50.

I now need regular monitoring and polyp removal. There is no cure, but proactive management, regular screening, a high-fibre diet, reducing processed foods, limiting alcohol and prioritising gut health can all help lower the risks. This diagnosis has been a wake-up call, reinforcing how vital it is to take ownership of our future health; nobody else will do it for you. I never thought this would be part of my journey, but I'm grateful it was caught early. Prevention isn't just important; it's essential for longevity and quality of life.

Women in the UK have access to several screening programmes, yet many of us don't fully take advantage of them. Why? Because we're busy? Because we're scared? Because we don't want to confront the what-ifs? Or we may not receive the letter inviting us. I get it. There's a psychological element to all of this. No one wants to think about cancer or chronic illness. But this approach puts us at far greater risk. Therefore, it is essential to understand our entitlements. Early detection is one of the most powerful tools for extending our lifespan and healthspan.

There's also a misconception that you don't need a check-up if you feel fine. However, many serious diseases are silent, especially in their early stages. High blood pressure and high cholesterol often do not present with noticeable symptoms. Additionally, cervical abnormalities usually exist without any noticeable signs. I've had conversations with women in my community who delayed their smear tests for years, only to finally go and be diagnosed with severe precancerous cells. One woman told me she was six months away from something far worse and that screening saved her life.

And did you know, heart disease is the leading cause of death for women in the UK – more than breast cancer?[14] However, because it's often considered a man's disease, many women don't realise they need to be proactive about their heart health. Routine health checks, including cholesterol and blood pressure screenings, can catch early warning signs before they lead to serious issues like heart attacks or strokes.

Here's the truth: no one will prioritise our health for us. Not our GP, not the NHS, not our families. The NHS offers several key screenings for women, including cervical smears, mammograms and bowel cancer tests, yet uptake is less than ideal. We have to be the ones to step up and take charge. That means:

- **Booking the appointments:** Stop putting off that smear test, mammogram or GP check-up.

- **Knowing our numbers:** Blood pressure, cholesterol and blood sugar levels matter, especially post-menopause.

- **Understanding our risk factors:** If you have a family history of breast cancer, heart disease or osteoporosis, you may need additional screenings.

- **Encouraging other women:** Discuss screenings with your friends, daughters and mothers. Fear thrives in silence, but support can make all the difference.

We can research the best diets, exercise routines and methods to boost longevity, but the simple, science-backed truth is this: early detection and prevention give us the best shot at a long, healthy life. The best-case scenario is that your screening comes back clear and you move forward with peace of mind. The second-best scenario? You catch something early enough to treat it effectively.

So, next time that letter from the NHS lands on your doormat, don't put it in the 'I'll deal with it later' pile. Take 5 minutes. Book the appointment. And remind yourself that prioritising screening is one of the greatest gifts you can give your future self. Prevention isn't just about living longer; it's about living better. And that's what true longevity is all about.

Cervical screening

- According to Cancer Research UK, cervical screening prevents an estimated 70% of cervical cancer deaths. If everyone attended, that number could jump to 83%. But attendance rates have dropped below 70% in some areas of England. Why? Many women put it off due to embarrassment, discomfort or simply not making the time.

- All women and people with a cervix between the ages of 25 and 64 should attend regular cervical screenings, with invitations sent by post. Screening frequency depends on age:
  - Those under 25 will receive an invitation up to 6 months before turning 25.
  - Individuals aged 25 to 49 are invited every 3 years, while those aged 50 to 64 are invited every 5 years.

- Screening is only offered after the age of 65 if a recent test result was abnormal. If you've missed a screening, you don't need to wait for another letter; you can book an appointment anytime. Screening schedules may vary across different parts of the UK; therefore, checking the guidelines for Scotland, Wales or Northern Ireland, as applicable, is essential.

- Cervical screening is not routinely offered to those under 25, as cervical cancer is rare in this age group and abnormal cell changes often resolve on their own.

- Similarly, screening stops after 65 unless there is a history of abnormal results, but those who have never been screened or haven't had one since 50 can request a test from their GP. If you've had a total hysterectomy (removal of the womb and cervix), cervical screening is no longer necessary, and you should not receive further invitations.[15]

Breast screening

The NHS Breast Screening Programme detects around 19,000 cancers each year, many at an early stage where treatment is far more effective. Women aged 50 to 70 are invited every 3 years, yet many decline. Again, fear and avoidance play a role.

- Anyone registered with a GP as female will be invited for NHS breast screening every 3 years between the ages of 50 and 71, and an invitation letter will be sent by post.

- The first invite is automatically sent between 50 and 53, followed by screenings every 3 years until 71.

- If you are a trans man, trans woman or non-binary, you may or may not be invited automatically, depending on how you are registered with your GP, so it's important to check with your GP surgery or local breast screening service if needed.

- You must be registered with a general practitioner (GP) to receive an invitation.

- If you have not received an invite by 53 and believe you should have, contact your local breast screening service. Those aged 71 and over will not be automatically invited, but can still request a screening every 3 years by contacting their local breast screening service.[16]

Bowel cancer screening

One of the deadliest cancers, bowel cancer, has a survival rate of over 90% if caught early.

- Bowel cancer screening is a free NHS test that you do at home, designed to check for signs of bowel cancer by looking for hidden blood in your stool using a faecal immunochemical test (FIT).

- It is offered every 2 years to everyone aged 54 to 74 and will soon be extended to include people aged 50 to 74.

- If you are over 75, you can still participate by calling the bowel cancer screening helpline on 0800 707 6060 to request a kit. The test involves collecting a small sample of your poo using the kit sent to your home, sealing it in the provided container, and posting it back in the envelope supplied – no stamp needed. You must be registered with a general practitioner (GP) and have a valid postal address to receive the kit automatically. However, you can also request that it be sent to an alternative address, including your GP surgery.

- If you've not received a test by the time you're 54 or think you're eligible but haven't been invited, you should contact the helpline. Results usually arrive within 2 weeks. Most people are told that no further tests are needed, but if blood is detected, you will be invited to speak with a specialist nurse and may be referred for a colonoscopy.

- Blood in the stool doesn't always mean cancer; it could be due to other issues like polyps or minor conditions such as fissures. Notably, while a negative result is reassuring, it doesn't rule out cancer completely, so staying aware of symptoms and speaking to your GP if anything changes is still vital. The screening process is optional, but it's one of the most effective tools for detecting bowel cancer early, often before any symptoms appear, making it easier to treat and significantly improving outcomes.

Each of these tests is quick and relatively non-invasive, and it could be the difference between catching something early and facing a far more difficult prognosis.

Other tests you could do that aren't routine check-ups

Bone health checks

Bone health is often overlooked until an issue arises and it is essential to note that the NHS does not routinely provide bone density testing, such as a DEXA scan. You will not be offered one during a standard check-up, despite its potential as an early warning sign for future problems.

That's why we need to be proactive. As someone diagnosed with osteopenia, I understand how easy it is to overlook this aspect of our health, especially when there are no apparent symptoms. However, I also recognise the importance of taking it seriously, particularly when considering the fall statistics for women in later life. Fragility fractures can entirely alter your independence and longevity.

As we move through menopause, protecting our bones is vital to safeguarding our long-term health. Around the average age of 51, oestrogen levels begin to decline, and with that comes an increased rate of bone loss. Oestrogen plays a key role in maintaining bone density, and studies show that up to 20% of bone loss can happen during the menopausal transition. Globally, one in ten women over 60 is affected by osteoporosis, a condition that weakens bones and increases their susceptibility to fractures.[17]

If you can access a DEXA scan privately or through your GP based on risk factors, it's a quick, painless way to check your bone density. However, this isn't always available unless you've had a fracture or meet specific criteria.

If you can't get a DEXA scan, I encourage you to ask your GP for a FRAX score instead. This clinical risk assessment, developed by the University of Sheffield, calculates your likelihood of fractures based on personal risk factors. It's a great starting point and something you can and should request if you've had unexplained fractures or are concerned about your bone health.

We don't need to wait for a break to take action. The sooner we understand and prioritise our bone health, the more empowered we become to live stronger, more mobile lives for longer.

Heart health checks

When it comes to heart health, women often get overlooked. After menopause, we lose much of the natural cardiovascular protection once provided by oestrogen. Despite this increased risk, heart screening isn't routinely offered to women in the same way that cervical or breast screening is. You are unlikely to be invited for a cardiovascular screening unless you are eligible for an NHS Health Check, which is offered every 5 years to people aged 40 to 74.

Unlike men, women are more likely to experience subtle symptoms of heart disease, such as fatigue, shortness of breath or indigestion-like discomfort, rather than the classic crushing chest pain. These symptoms are easily mistaken for stress or anxiety, leading to frequent misdiagnosis or underdiagnosis.

Cholesterol also becomes an essential factor to monitor as we age. While our bodies need some cholesterol to function well, having too much, especially LDL (often called 'bad' cholesterol), can put your circulation under pressure. Over time, this can lead to the build-up of fatty deposits in the arteries. If a blockage forms and stops blood flow to the heart or brain, it can trigger serious events such as angina, heart attacks or strokes.

A simple blood test to check your cholesterol levels is a valuable tool. It not only gives you a snapshot of your cardiovascular risk but can also serve as the nudge you need to make empowering changes, whether adjusting your diet, moving more regularly or rethinking stress and sleep habits.

It's crucial to be proactive. If you have risk factors like a family history of heart disease, high blood pressure, high cholesterol, diabetes, smoking or are going through menopause, speak to your GP and ask for a heart health check, even if you feel fine. And if you're experiencing unexplained fatigue, breathlessness or discomfort, don't ignore it.

Blood pressure tests

Up to 66% of men and 71% of women aged 75 and over have high blood pressure, but many don't realise it as they often have no symptoms.[18]

Blood pressure is the force that your blood exerts on the walls of your arteries. Common symptoms of low blood pressure include nausea and dizziness. High blood pressure, however, rarely has noticeable symptoms but can weaken your heart and damage the walls of your arteries, increasing the risk of heart disease, stroke and kidney disease.

Your pharmacist, practice nurse or GP will use a cuff that fits around your upper arm and is inflated until it becomes tight. The test is quick, painless and only takes a minute. You can even buy a monitor to use at home. If your results fall outside the normal range, you must have them checked several more times. If your blood pressure is consistently found to be high, your GP will discuss with you how to lower it. If your blood pressure is low, your GP may suggest lifestyle changes, such as drinking more water, to help raise it.

You may be offered a blood test to assess the functioning of your kidneys and another test to evaluate your risk of developing diabetes. Treatment may include lifestyle changes, and if these aren't successful or your blood pressure is very high, you're likely to be prescribed medication.

Skin checks

Whether you check yourself or visit a specialist clinic, monitoring moles can help you spot the early signs of skin cancer. Most moles are harmless, but sometimes they can develop into a rare form of skin cancer called malignant melanoma.

You should check for new moles every few weeks and see your doctor if you notice a change in an existing mole's colour, size or shape. Ask your GP to examine it and, if necessary, refer you for further testing. A specialist may recommend its removal. If it's found to be melanoma, you may need additional tests to check that the cancer has not spread.

Melanoma is the fifth most common cancer in the UK, with around 16,700 new cases diagnosed each year, and as with all cancers, early detection and treatment increase your chances of surviving it.[19]

CHAPTER 4

The Role of Female Hormones in Ageing

Hormones are central to a woman's health throughout her entire lifespan. Shifts in hormones from puberty to pregnancy, and then through menopause and postmenopause, have a significant impact on mental health, physical well-being, metabolism, bone density, cardiovascular function and other aspects of health.

During puberty, rising levels of oestrogen and progesterone establish the reproductive system, while also affecting mood, energy levels and metabolic function. Pregnancy and the postpartum period involve significant hormonal changes, shaping long-term physical and emotional health.

However, it is during midlife, through the transition from perimenopause into postmenopause, that hormonal changes most significantly impact future health risks. Oestrogen, a hormone that protects many systems in the body, declines sharply during this period. This decline is linked to increased risks of cardiovascular disease, osteoporosis, type 2 diabetes and cognitive decline. We will explore these risks further as we move through the key health pillars later in this book. But first, it is essential to understand the stages of hormonal change and their implications.

Perimenopause

Perimenopause is the phase leading up to menopause, where hormone levels, particularly oestrogen and progesterone, begin to fluctuate and decline. This stage often starts between the ages of 45 and 55, although it can occur earlier. In the UK, the average age for menopause is 51. Early menopause affects around one in 100 women before the age of 40, and one in 1,000 women before 30.[20]

Currently, around 13 million women in the UK are experiencing some stage of menopause, highlighting how common and important it is to understand this transition.

Perimenopause brings a wide range of symptoms, of which over 60 have been recognised. The most common include:

- hot flushes
- mood changes, including anxiety and depression
- sleep disturbances and insomnia
- fatigue and low energy
- irregular or heavier periods
- joint aches and pains

These symptoms can significantly disrupt daily life and, if not effectively managed, may lead to a decline in physical activity, poor sleep quality and unhealthy eating patterns, factors that negatively impact long-term health and longevity.

However, symptoms are manageable. As I discussed in *Owning Your Menopause: Fitter, Calmer, Stronger in 30 Days*, targeted lifestyle strategies such as strength training, optimal nutrition, improving sleep hygiene, and mental well-being practices can help women feel more in control and better support their long-term health.

Menopause: A Defined Moment

Despite the many changes leading up to it, menopause itself refers to a single day: the point at which twelve consecutive months have passed without a menstrual period. It marks the official end of reproductive capacity. After menopause, the body enters a new hormonal environment, with significantly reduced ovarian oestrogen and progesterone production.

Postmenopause: The New Normal

Postmenopause begins the day after menopause and continues for the rest of a woman's life. Hormone levels remain low during this time. The body produces a weaker form of oestrogen called oestrone, mainly through fat tissue. This shift can alter body composition, often increasing fat storage around the abdomen. Importantly, this is not just a cosmetic concern. Increased abdominal fat is associated with a higher risk of insulin resistance, type 2 diabetes, cardiovascular disease and certain types of cancer.

The decline in oestrogen also removes a layer of protection for bones and the cardiovascular system, raising the risk of osteoporosis and heart disease.[21]

These changes are significant but not inevitable. Interventions such as strength training, mindful nutrition, quality sleep and stress management can profoundly impact health outcomes in postmenopause. This is the foundation for the 21-Day Plan outlined later in this book.

HRT

Hormone replacement therapy (HRT) can be an effective way to manage the symptoms of menopause and protect long-term health. Despite fears that arose from earlier studies, current evidence shows that for many women, particularly those under 60 or within 10 years of menopause, HRT can be both safe and beneficial.[22]

HRT can:

- reduce hot flushes, mood swings and sleep disturbances
- preserve bone density and lower fracture risk
- support cardiovascular health
- potentially protect cognitive function and reduce the risk of dementia

However, HRT is not a universal solution. It should be personalised, with type, dosage and delivery method tailored to individual needs and health history. It is essential to work with a healthcare provider experienced in menopause management to determine the best course of action.

It is also essential to view HRT as one part of a broader approach. Lifestyle strategies such as strength training, healthy eating, adequate sleep and stress management remain critical, regardless of whether HRT is used. HRT can support the transition through menopause, but it cannot replace the foundations of good health.

The Hormones Involved in Menopause

Here are the leading hormonal players and how they change during the menopause transition.

> **Oestrogen**
> Oestrogen is the most well-known hormone related to menopause, and for good reason. It's responsible for:
> - Regulating the menstrual cycle
> - Supporting bone density
> - Maintaining healthy cholesterol levels
> - Keeping the vaginal tissues and bladder healthy
> - Supporting mood and cognitive function
> - Helping regulate body temperature
>
> During perimenopause, **oestrogen begins to fluctuate wildly**, causing many of the common symptoms like hot flushes, mood swings and irregular periods. Eventually, levels **drop dramatically** as the ovaries slow and stop hormone production. This long-term deficiency is what contributes to many postmenopausal health risks like **osteoporosis**, **heart disease** and **changes in body composition**.
>
> Oestrogen doesn't just switch off, it tapers off, sometimes erratically. This can feel like an emotional and physical rollercoaster.

Progesterone

Often referred to as the balancing hormone, progesterone works in harmony with oestrogen and is key for:
- Regulating mood
- Supporting sleep
- Reducing anxiety
- Preparing the uterus for pregnancy
- Maintaining a regular menstrual cycle

During perimenopause, **progesterone is often the first hormone to start declining**, which can lead to:
- Irregular or heavy periods
- Increased anxiety and irritability
- Poor sleep
- A sense of feeling 'wired but tired'

Testosterone

Many people are surprised to learn that women also produce testosterone – in smaller amounts than men, of course, but still important for:
- Supporting libido
- Maintaining muscle mass and strength
- Boosting confidence and motivation
- Aiding cognitive function (especially focus and drive)

Testosterone production gradually declines with age and may dip more noticeably during or after menopause. Some women find their **energy, confidence** and **sexual desire** shift as a result.

CHAPTER 5

Redefining Ageing

For generations, society has framed ageing for women as a process of decline, a loss of beauty, energy, relevance and purpose. Ageing has often been portrayed as an inevitable descent into invisibility, where women are expected to fade into the background quietly. This narrative, repeated across decades, has left many women feeling anxious, inadequate and resistant towards a completely natural and universal part of life. I know this perception shaped my views growing up and, without question, it influenced how I once visualised ageing.

While we are beginning to see positive change, the widespread availability of aesthetic solutions, which were previously accessible only to those who could afford them, can create the illusion that acceptance is more widespread than it truly is. Our society still struggles to view ageing, especially for women, through a lens of vitality and opportunity.

It is worth asking: why is ageing viewed so differently between men and women? Ageing in men is often framed positively, associated with terms like Silver Fox, suggesting sophistication, wisdom and enduring appeal. However, the language tends to diminish for women: over the hill, old maid or, even when meant to be flattering, patronising labels like granny chic. Nothing highlights this double standard more than the phrase, 'You look good for your age,' an offhand comment that begs the question: what exactly is someone my age supposed to look like?

This mindset around ageing is deeply flawed. It is rooted not only in the fear of physical decline but also in the fear of losing health, identity and value. For women, these fears are compounded by the immense societal pressure to prioritise appearance over substance. Marketing terms like 'anti-ageing' reinforce the damaging belief that growing older is something to be resisted rather than something to be embraced, nurtured and optimised.

These outdated narratives affect self-esteem and have real consequences for health and longevity. Women who internalise these messages may become less likely to invest in themselves just when their bodies and minds need proactive support the most. When we associate ageing solely with decline, we risk giving up habits that can extend and enrich our lives.

Changing this narrative is essential for emotional well-being, physical health, resilience and longevity. How we perceive ageing directly influences how we move through it. Those who approach ageing with a sense of possibility, purpose and proactive self-care live longer, healthier lives. Research consistently shows that a positive attitude towards ageing is linked to better cardiovascular health, stronger cognitive function and greater longevity.[23]

We have an extraordinary opportunity to redefine ageing for ourselves. Rather than seeing it as a loss, we can see it as an evolution where strength, mobility, vitality and connection are maintained and enhanced. By nurturing our bodies through movement, strength-building exercises, good nutrition, restorative sleep and mental well-being practices, we can maintain our youthfulness where it matters most: energy, spirit and capability.

The future of ageing is not about resisting change but about embracing it with strength, intention and optimism.

Ageing as an Opportunity

I would love women to see that ageing is not about decline but transformation; it's a powerful and empowering life stage full of opportunities to grow, thrive and live authentically.

Age brings an unmatched depth of experience. The challenges and triumphs over decades create profound wisdom and resilience, enabling older adults to approach life with confidence and grace that only comes with time. For women, in particular, ageing can be a time to shed societal expectations and embrace their true selves. With life experience comes a greater understanding of what truly matters, allowing them to navigate life with renewed clarity and purpose. As I age, I worry less about what people think. 'Those that mind don't matter, and those that matter don't mind' is something I take into my days. Equally, I have carved out a new career in my forties and see this as just the beginning; I am excited for the next chapter of my life. Bringing my life wisdom into my job has been valuable, enabling me to empathise more with my clients.

The misconception that ageing is synonymous with illness must be challenged. While health changes as we age, it is possible to thrive physically, mentally and emotionally in later years. Strength training, balanced nutrition, restorative sleep and mindfulness practices can help people maintain energy and vitality well into their last decades.

Let's celebrate this chapter of life as a time of possibility, power and fulfilment.

CHAPTER 6

Relationships and Their Impact on Health and Longevity

I don't know about you, but I've found that relationships with family and my partner have become increasingly complex as I've aged. Don't get me wrong, there are many joyful and rewarding moments. However, the demands of work, caregiving, parenting adult children, managing perimenopause and trying to maintain a loving partnership have created stress that has taken a toll on both my mental and physical well-being. This is one of the many reasons this book is significant for me. I want to help others navigate these challenges with greater ease, understanding and compassion.

Understanding relationship dynamics, forgiving ourselves and adopting strategies to maintain balance are crucial for preserving our overall well-being, happiness and longevity.

Caring for ageing or ill parents is a profound responsibility many midlife women face. I cared for my father during the last 18 months of his life as he battled pancreatic cancer. Watching him decline was heartbreaking. The weight of responsibility, late-night worries and the constant juggling between his care and the rest of life's demands were overwhelming. Family tensions often surfaced as we navigated difficult decisions, and I frequently questioned whether I was doing enough for everyone.

Caregiving isn't just emotionally draining; it's also physically demanding. It can involve lifting, assisting or moving a loved one, all while running on little sleep and neglecting your own needs. I skipped meals, pushed through exhaustion and brushed aside my well-being. It wasn't sustainable.

Eventually, I realised I couldn't do it all alone. Asking for help from my husband and friends wasn't a weakness but a necessity. Sharing the load made a world of difference.

Setting realistic expectations and acknowledging our limits are essential for managing caregiving stress. Prioritising sleep, regular movement and nourishing food helps sustain the energy we need. Whether from friends, counsellors or support groups, emotional support offers a safe space to share, reflect and receive practical advice. These aren't luxuries. They're vital tools for coping without losing ourselves, but for some reason, many women struggle with asking for help.

As my kids have grown into adults, my parenting role has shifted. I'm no longer part of their daily routines, but I offer emotional and financial support. This phase has its challenges. I've had to learn how to maintain strong relationships while being clear about boundaries and expectations.

There's been a learning curve for me, my husband and the kids. I want them to take ownership of their lives, even though watching them make mistakes is difficult. At the same time, I've had to be honest about what I can and cannot give, whether that's time, money or emotional bandwidth, so I don't feel overwhelmed or resentful.

Open communication is key. It helps prevent misunderstandings and ensures we're all on the same page. While this stage of parenting is different, it presents an opportunity to nurture balanced and fulfilling relationships with our adult children.

Many of my friends have experienced a loss of identity after their children left home, often referred to as 'empty nest syndrome'. Others have encountered the unexpected stress of adult children moving back in due to financial or personal struggles or even taking on caregiving roles for their grandchildren. These changes can be challenging, especially when combined with the hormonal and emotional shifts of menopause.

Midlife transitions often place pressure on long-term relationships. Hormonal fluctuations can lead to mood swings, decreased libido or fatigue, which may create emotional distance. At the same time, partners may face ageing-related challenges, career shifts or retirement, which can add to the strain. Caregiving responsibilities, whether for children, grandchildren or ageing parents, also often leave little time or energy for nurturing our partnerships.

Rebuilding and maintaining connections takes effort and intention. Honest conversations, shared journalling and simply carving out time to reflect together can bring couples closer. Acknowledging each other's needs and viewing change as an opportunity to grow, rather than a threat, can help deepen intimacy and connection.

With all these roles of carer, parent and partner, it becomes easy for women to put their own needs last. But neglecting ourselves only leads to burnout and health issues. To show up for others, we must first show up for ourselves.

That's why the practices in the 21-Day habit reset, like journalling, mindfulness, movement and setting boundaries, are so essential. They're not extras. They're the foundations for building resilience, protecting your health and feeling more grounded with life's shifting demands.

While many experiences I've shared reflect my journey as a mother, daughter and partner, I want to acknowledge that midlife looks different for everyone. Whether you're single, child-free, part of the LGBTQ+ community, a solo parent, navigating blended families or in a non-traditional partnership, midlife still presents unique challenges and changes that can impact your relationships and sense of identity.

Single and solo parents

For those raising children alone by choice, circumstance or through separation, there is often no one to share the daily responsibilities with. The physical and emotional load can be relentless, especially when paired with the symptoms of perimenopause or caregiving for older family members. Without a partner to lean on, solo parents often feel the pressure to hold it all together and may neglect their own needs entirely. Prioritising support networks, such as friends, community groups or professionals, is not just helpful, it's essential for sustainability.

LGBTQ+

LGBTQ+ individuals can face additional layers of complexity in their relationships. They may have experienced estrangement from their families and can have fewer legal protections in caregiving roles and limited access to inclusive healthcare, especially around menopause and ageing. For midlife LGBTQ+ people in long-term relationships, navigating changes in identity, libido or body image can feel isolating if not openly discussed. And for those who've chosen not to or have been unable to have children, concerns about future caregiving or loneliness in later life can emerge sharply.

Creating safe spaces for open conversation and seeking out affirming communities or therapists can make a world of difference. Everyone deserves to be supported in a way that respects their identity and values.[24]

Child-free by choice or circumstance

Not everyone becomes a parent and that decision or outcome can carry its emotional complexity in midlife. Some experience a profound sense of peace, freedom and autonomy. Others may confront societal assumptions or unspoken grief about what might have been. When friends focus on their adult children or grandchildren, those who are child-free can sometimes feel like they are observing from the outside.

Midlife, however, can also be a powerful time to explore legacy in a broader sense, such as mentoring, creating, leading or simply nurturing one's chosen family and community. The value we bring to others isn't limited to biology.

Blended families and step-parenting (a personal reflection)

Blending families in midlife isn't just about forming new connections; it's often about navigating old wounds, unspoken loyalties and roles that aren't always chosen but fall into our laps when life changes unexpectedly. I have first-hand experience of this.

As my father became seriously ill, I stepped into a caregiving role that was emotionally and physically intense. However, the family dynamic in my blended family was already complicated. Past resentments, unresolved tensions and unclear boundaries made the situation even more difficult and painful. I found myself not only managing his declining health but also trying to hold together a fragile web of relationships, some of which didn't always feel welcoming or supportive.

There were moments when I questioned my place, even as I devoted so much of myself. The emotional burden of watching my father decline was already heavy. Still, specific family dynamics left me feeling isolated and torn between doing what felt right for him and navigating the expectations and sometimes resentments others had towards my actions.

This experience opened my eyes to the profound complexity of blended families, especially during times of crisis. Our roles don't always align with how others perceive us and that mismatch can be hurtful. What helped me was acknowledging that I couldn't control how others behaved, only how I showed up with integrity, love and care for my well-being.

Blended families may never feel tidy or straightforward. Yet, they don't have to be perfect to be meaningful. Sometimes, the greatest strength lies in showing compassion, even when challenging, and recognising that your story, your effort and your place in the family matter, even if they aren't always acknowledged in the way you desire.

Caring for chosen family or friends

Not everyone has a traditional family structure. For many, close friends *are* their family. This sometimes means stepping into a caregiving role for a friend rather than a relative or relying on friends for support during illness or crisis. These relationships can be just as deep and meaningful, yet societal norms or systems often do not acknowledge or support them.

It is essential to recognise and validate the emotional weight of these connections. Caregiving deserves respect, and those who do it must prioritise their well-being.

Regardless of your relationship status, family structure or background, midlife transitions require something from you. Therefore, protecting your health, managing stress and maintaining connections with yourself and others is essential. You deserve support that meets you where you are and habits that help you thrive during and beyond your unique midlife experience.

PART 2
The Three Pillars of Longevity for Women

Before truly understanding what the word meant to me and writing this book, longevity conjured up images of ultra-marathon runners, biohacking billionaires and green-juice-drinking gurus defying the years. I have since learnt, and this is what I want to share with you, that true longevity, the kind that keeps you mobile, independent, joyful and mentally sharp well into your later decades, doesn't come from magic pills, expensive gadgets or extreme routines. It comes from the everyday choices we make. Those choices don't have to be overwhelming, complicated or inaccessible. They're often beautifully simple.

Movement, Nutrition and Mental Well-being. When you focus on strengthening these areas, you're not just improving how you show up today, you're building the strength, vitality and resilience that will carry you into a longer, healthier life. Everything changes when you start working with your body instead of feeling like it's fighting against you. You step into a new level of confidence, energy and freedom.

And alongside these pillars, there's something else I've found to be just as powerful: journalling.

Writing down how you feel, what you're noticing and what's working gives you a space to slow down and check in with yourself. It connects the dots between the physical changes you're experiencing and the emotional landscape that so often gets ignored. Journalling helps you become more mindful of your habits and patterns, and it's where you'll often spot the real breakthroughs happening. It's not about writing a perfect diary, it's about tuning into your own life as it unfolds. When you bring this kind of awareness to the changes you're making, you create a deeper sense of purpose and ownership over your health journey. You start to feel less like a passive participant and more like the expert on your own body, which you absolutely are.

I completely get it if this sounds like a lot to take in. There's a lot of overwhelming advice: do this, don't do that, eat this, avoid that. It can feel like you need to change everything all at once, and this is where many of us quit or don't feel like we can maintain the new habits we want to adopt. That's why I'm keeping it simple. Instead of bombarding you with a never-ending list of health rules, I want you to focus on just the three key pillars and your journal, which will become a powerful ally as you go.

- **Movement:** Essential because it builds the foundation for strength, flexibility and mobility, supporting independence and longevity.

- **Nutrition:** Primarily plant-based, this is vital because you are what you eat. Nutritious food powers every function in your body.

- **Mental well-being:** Connection and community are crucial because your mindset, stress levels and emotional resilience are just as essential as physical health.

And journalling threads all of this together. It's the reflection piece that helps you see what's shifting, what matters most and where to go next.

This isn't about quick fixes or overhauling your life overnight. It's about real, sustainable habits that will help you feel stronger, more energised and more in control of your body and mind. We'll do it together, step by step, with a 21-Day Plan designed to help you feel amazing without being overwhelmed, regardless of your starting point.

PART 2.1
Movement

Forget punishing workouts and unrealistic fitness goals. When it comes to longevity, movement is about function, not aesthetics. Our ability to move confidently, without pain or fear of falling, becomes one of the most significant predictors of how well we'll age.

As we age, we naturally lose muscle and joint mobility, but this doesn't have to be a downhill slide.[25] With targeted movements focused on stability and mobility, you can improve balance, maintain coordination, strengthen your core and protect your joints and bones.

This isn't about lifting the heaviest weights or training for marathons; it's about moving with intention. Consider incorporating resistance training, bodyweight exercises, functional movement patterns and low-impact activities, such as walking, Pilates and yoga, into your life. These tools, which you will learn in this book, help you with what may seem like the easiest of tasks at the moment – climbing stairs, getting up off the floor without assistance and feeling confident in your body – for years to come.

Longevity thrives in a body that can move freely, safely and with joy.

CHAPTER 7

Staying Strong and Independent

Many people start to notice changes in their bodies at some point in midlife. For me, it was a clear and undeniable wake-up call. Energy levels dropped. Minor aches and stiffness appeared. Clothes felt tighter. These signs were small but persistent reminders that my body was changing.

In that moment, I realised something needed to shift. I didn't want to continue feeling this way and knew action was necessary. If you recognise that feeling, this chapter is for you.

Regular exercise is one of the most powerful tools to extend our lifespan, healthspan and the quality of life we enjoy as we age. The statistics are sobering, though. One in three women aged 41 to 60 in the UK isn't meeting the recommended 150 minutes of exercise per week. One in five is doing less than 30 minutes. Women are living, on average, nearly 20 years in poor health. That's two decades during which many of us are surviving, not thriving. But it doesn't have to be that way.[26]

Studies consistently show that people who remain physically active reduce their risk of chronic conditions like heart disease, diabetes, stroke and some cancers. They also experience improved mood, sharper cognitive function and overall mobility.

Movement is not just helpful for ageing well, it is essential. However, not all types of exercise offer the same benefits. To build lasting strength, resilience and confidence in the years ahead, it is essential to focus on three key areas:

Aerobic (cardiovascular) fitness, anaerobic (strength) training and flexibility and mobility exercises. Each supports the body in different but equally important ways:

- **Aerobic activities:** Walking, dancing, swimming and cycling enhance heart and lung function, boost circulation and help regulate weight. According to NHS guidelines, adults should aim for at least 150 minutes of moderate-intensity or 75 minutes of vigorous-intensity aerobic activity each week.

- **Equally important is anaerobic strength training:** As muscle mass naturally declines with age, incorporating weightlifting, resistance band exercises and bodyweight exercises becomes essential. Strength training helps preserve joint health, supports metabolic function and maintains the ability to perform daily tasks. It's a non-negotiable for physical independence and overall vitality, and just two sessions per week can make a significant difference.

- **Lastly, flexibility and mobility are often overlooked:** Yet they are central to longevity. That's why they're a core part of the 21-Day Plan. These practices help reduce stiffness, improve range of motion and enhance coordination and balance, protecting you against falls and helping you stay agile as the years pass.

Beyond the physical benefits, exercise is crucial to mental and emotional well-being. Movement triggers the release of endorphins, which help elevate mood and reduce stress. It also supports brain health by increasing brain-derived neurotrophins, proteins that promote cognitive function and help protect against conditions like Alzheimer's. Regular physical activity also reduces inflammation and oxidative stress, which contribute to cellular ageing, and encourages repair at the deepest level.

Consistency is where the magic happens: sustainable, enjoyable habits. Even short, manageable sessions, like a 10-minute walk, can spark change. Movement adapts to every stage of life, and its benefits ripple across every dimension of your health. When you move purposefully, you invest in a future filled with energy, independence and joy.

Movement for Longevity

In the following sections, we'll explain each type of movement and how you can apply it to your life practically and sustainably. I've also included a table that organises exercises into these three categories to help you implement this.

Aerobic exercise

Aerobic exercise is what most of us think of as the cardio part of exercise, which gets your heart beating faster, your breath a little shorter, and your body warmer.

Aerobic exercise strengthens your cardiovascular system, supports metabolism and improves your workouts and everyday life endurance.[27] Moreover, it helps regulate blood pressure, balance blood sugar and support brain function. It's also an excellent mood booster; thanks to endorphins and rhythmic movement, it can alleviate anxiety, clear brain fog and improve sleep quality.

But don't worry, it doesn't have to mean pounding the pavement or sweating buckets in a spin class unless that's your thing. Aerobic exercise simply means moving in a way that gets your heart and lungs working for an extended period. Walking up the stairs without getting out of breath? Dancing at a wedding and not needing to sit down after two songs? That's aerobic fitness.

I started working with a woman who, at 52, realised she had begun avoiding hills on her daily dog walks because they left her breathless. We talked, and not only did she start strength training with me, but I encouraged her to add 10 minutes of brisk walking after dinner – nothing fancy, no trainers, no apps. Within a few weeks, those hills didn't feel so daunting. She gradually increased her pace, added some gentle jogging intervals, and, as I write this, is considering the Three Peaks Challenge. Not only that, but her blood pressure decreased, her sleep improved and, most importantly, she felt proud of her body again.

You don't need to run to get the benefits. Fast-paced walking, swimming, dancing around your kitchen, gardening or cycling all count. If it raises your heart rate, and you're moving steadily for 10 minutes or more, it's doing your body good.

Please remember that walking briskly for 30 minutes can be just as beneficial, particularly when done consistently. Movement doesn't have to be punishing to be effective, and sweat is not the measure of success. What truly matters is your heart rate, how you feel, and that you're moving your body purposefully.

Anaerobic exercise

Anaerobic exercise builds strength, power and muscle, often boosting metabolism more after exercise than aerobic activities. If there's one form of anaerobic exercise that every woman should embrace in midlife, it's strength training. This may feel the most intimidating, especially if you've never touched a weight. But bear with me, because this type of movement is a game-changer.

Strength or resistance training is any movement that uses force to engage your muscles. This can be achieved with weights, resistance bands, or even your body weight. I will elaborate on why we train this way: to build and maintain lean muscle mass, support your bones, improve your posture, and keep your metabolism functioning optimally.

After the age of 30, we naturally lose muscle every decade, a process that accelerates during menopause.[28] If we don't actively train to keep it, we lose it. That means more than just feeling weaker; it affects how much energy we burn at rest, how well we move and even how stable we are on our feet.

I have already shared my experience of my mum starting resistance exercising at 76, but I only started myself at 40. I was researching exercise due to my chronic aches and pains, not yet realising I was in perimenopause, and everything pointed towards lifting weights. Looking back, much of the pain was inflammation from doing too much HIIT. This doesn't mean you should avoid this kind of exercise; instead, it means please do it with an understanding that it can elevate stress in the body, and switching can be beneficial, not detrimental, for a period of time. Come back to it when you feel ready.

One of the most significant aspects of strength training is its sense of empowerment. Lifting something heavy, according to your standards, not anyone else's, signals to your brain that you are strong, capable and resilient.

Strength training is a form of anaerobic exercise because it relies on quick, intense bursts of effort powered by energy stored in your muscles, rather than oxygen. These short bouts, typically lasting from just a few seconds to around 2 minutes, include activities such as lifting weights, short bursts of fast running, bodyweight circuits and high-intensity intervals (HIIT).

This is also a good opportunity to dispel a myth that has persisted far too long. YOU WON'T GET BULKY. Women typically do not have the hormone levels to naturally 'bulk up' without significant effort.[29] Instead, you will get stronger, more defined muscles and a powerful sense of confidence.

Also, please note that it is never too late to start strength training. Studies have shown that individuals in their seventies, eighties and even nineties can gain muscle mass and improve their function through resistance training.

Aerobic vs Anaerobic Exercise

Feature	Aerobic Exercise	Anaerobic Exercise
Energy Source	Oxygen	Stored energy in muscles (glycogen)
Duration	Long, sustained (minutes to hours)	Short bursts (seconds to 2 minutes)
Intensity	Moderate	High to very high
Examples	Walking, jogging, swimming, dancing	Sprinting, HIIT, weightlifting, jump squats
Primary Benefit	Cardiovascular endurance, fat burning	Muscle building, power, speed, metabolism boost
Breathing	Deep, steady breathing	Rapid, heavy breathing
Recovery Time	Shorter	Longer (more rest needed between sets)

Flexibility and mobility

This is the most overlooked and underrated type of movement, but in my eyes, it's the glue that holds everything else together. Flexibility and mobility enable us to navigate life easily, comfortably and confidently.

Flexibility refers to the ability of your muscles and tendons to stretch, while mobility relates to how freely and efficiently your joints move. Together, they influence your ability to perform activities we often take for granted until they become more challenging, such as reaching, bending, twisting and balancing.

If you've ever groaned getting out of bed or noticed it's trickier to reach the top shelf than it used to be, you've felt the effects of lost mobility.

Mobility and flexibility work doesn't need to be long or complicated. A few simple daily stretches, dynamic warm-ups before walks or workouts, and the occasional yoga or Pilates class, can significantly improve your body's overall feel.

Think of flexibility like hydration; your body will thank you whenever you do it. Stretching and mobility exercises are essential for injury prevention, maintaining joint health and promoting functional movement as we age.

The key to movement is to find a rhythm that works for you, a balance of heart-healthy movement, strength-building work and gentle, nourishing mobility practice. Think of your body like a home: cardio strengthens the plumbing, strength builds the walls and flexibility keeps the doors and windows moving smoothly.

Overleaf is a table I've put together to illustrate the various ways you can bring this plan to life through movement. Whether you prefer walking, strength training, dancing or stretching, there's something here for everyone. This isn't about perfection, it's about finding activities that you enjoy and that fit into your real life. Use this table as inspiration to shape your routine in a way that feels good, supports your goals and keeps you coming back for more.

Ways of Exercising and Benefits

Types of Movement	Benefits	To Note
Anaerobic Exercise		
Lifting weights	• Builds and maintains muscle mass • Strengthens bones • Helps joint flexibility • Creates mobility • Builds self-confidence • Controls blood sugar • Decreases risk of falls • Lowers the risk of injury • Improves heart health • Boosts mood • Improves brain health • Lowers the risk of high blood pressure • Suitable for any level and age • Boosts the immune system	Start gradually and always ensure you know your form to avoid injury. Invest in some good, sturdy dumbbells. Warm up and cool down. Allow time between your sessions so your muscles can be repaired.
HIIT (High-Intensity Interval Training)	• Quick • Improves stamina • Can increase strength • Good for your heart • Helps regulate blood sugar • Lowers the risk of high blood pressure • Boosts mood	TOO MUCH HIIT can elevate your cortisol levels, which can have a negative impact on a menopausal woman. I suggest 1–2 sessions a week MAX.
Spin	• Kinder on joints • Good for endurance	Be mindful of the amount you do, as can raise cortisol levels. It is a great way to meet people and the music can really boost your endorphins.

Aerobic exercise		
LISS (Low-Intensity Steady State) Cardio	• Suitable for all levels • Lowers the risk of high blood pressure • Kinder on joints • Good for endurance • Suitable for a recovery session • Boosts mood • Boosts the immune system	LISS is great but requires more time, 45–60 minutes. It's great if you are doing endurance events. You could get bored, so mix up your LISS with walking, cycling, swimming and jogging.
Walking	• Suitable for all levels and ages • For all the family • Lowers the risk of high blood pressure • Kinder on joints • Good for endurance • Suitable for a recovery session • Great for your mental health • Free • Readily possible • Boosts mood • Boosts the immune system	It is important to ensure you add some strength training sessions alongside your walks to maximise your fitness plan's benefits.
Anaerobic and aerobic exercise		
Running	• Can help manage stress • Free • Suitable for all ages and levels • Great for heart and lung health • Helps balance sugar levels • Boosts mood • Boosts the immune system	Incorporate strength training alongside your running, especially to help with recovery and endurance. If you are experiencing aches and pains, it's okay to rest and recover and come back to it when you are up for the challenge.

Dance	• Improves heart health • Can help with strength and endurance • Increases your aerobic fitness • Helps with coordination, agility and flexibility • Music can help with mood • Free • Suitable for all levels and ages • Boosts immune system	Going to a dance class, dancing at home or on a night out is a mood-booster and can build self-confidence.
Cycling	• Can help manage stress • Free • Kinder on joints • Good for endurance • It's suitable for all ages and levels, and a great family activity • Great for heart and lung health • Helps balance sugar levels • Boosts mood • Boosts immune system	Try to incorporate strength training alongside your cycling, especially to help with endurance and balance.
Flexibility and mobility		
Pilates	• Helps relieve tension • Promotes body awareness • Kinder on joints • Builds muscle, balance, stability and mobility • Improves flexibility • Increases core strength • Decreases back pain • Improves posture • Suitable for all levels and ages • Boosts mood • Boosts immune system	Pilates is a great addition to a programme as we go through menopause and midlife. It will help with recovery and can be a wonderful option for many who are experiencing joint aches and pains.

Yoga	• Helps relieve tension • Improves breathing • Kinder on joints • Builds muscle, balance, stability and mobility • Improves flexibility • Increases core strength • Decreases back pain • Improves posture • Suitable for all levels and ages • Boosts mood • Boosts immune system	Yoga is a great addition to a programme as we go through menopause and midlife. It will help with recovery and can be a wonderful option for many who are experiencing joint aches and pains. It can help you to focus more on your breath, which can benefit overall health and well-being
Barre	• Helps relieve tension • Promotes body awareness • Kinder on joints • Builds muscle, balance, stability and mobility • Improves flexibility • Increases core strength • Decreases back pain • Improves posture • Suitable for all levels and ages • Boosts mood • Boosts the immune system	You will likely need to invest in some bands, low weights and have a stable chair to perform some of the moves.

Of course, there are other opportunities and ways to move the body for those who are time-poor, and excellent evidence-based research suggests that 'exercise snacking' can have some benefits.

Exercise snacking

Imagine if, when you felt time-poor and were struggling to carve out any time for the gym, you could break your movement into manageable bites throughout the day. No change of clothes, no commute, no stress. Just quick bursts of movement: a few squats while the kettle boils, a brisk stair climb after a Zoom call or a 1-minute plank while dinner simmers. That's the beauty of exercise snacking, and it's also fast becoming a powerful longevity tool. However, it should not be seen as a replacement for longer chunks of movement, which are fundamental. It is a time-saving strategy on the days you are pushed.

The idea is simple: movement doesn't have to be long or structured to be effective. These 'snacks' of exercise can be as short as 1–5 minutes long, repeated a few times a day, and yet pack a powerful punch. They can elevate your heart rate, build strength, improve balance and even enhance insulin sensitivity. And most importantly, they're doable. Which, in midlife, might just be the secret ingredient to staying consistent.

Researchers at Leeds Beckett University have explored the concept of exercise snacking. Their findings suggest that this approach can be particularly effective in managing blood glucose levels, providing a practical strategy for individuals with, or at risk of, type 2 diabetes.[30]

A scoping review published in *Sports Medicine* in 2024 examined various studies on exercise snacking. The review concluded that brief, intermittent bouts of physical activity are associated with reduced morbidity and mortality, particularly in relation to cardiovascular health. The authors emphasised the feasibility and safety of exercise snacks, noting their potential to improve cardiorespiratory fitness and overall health.[31]

The beauty of exercise snacking lies in how it mimics our ancestral patterns of frequent functional movement scattered throughout the day. Our bodies thrive on this kind of intermittent loading. When you move regularly in short bursts, you keep your muscles activated, your blood flowing and your metabolism ticking – all essential for preventing age-related decline.

These micro-movements also help:

- Maintain and build muscle mass, especially if strength training is involved (such as squats or press-ups).

- Improve mobility and joint health, which helps prevent falls and injuries.

- Boost mitochondrial function, which supports energy production and cellular health, and is crucial for ageing well.

- Break up sedentary time, which research shows is an independent risk factor for chronic diseases, regardless of your gym time.

Consistency trumps intensity. Exercise snacking makes consistency more achievable, especially on hectic days when a full workout feels impossible. And for women navigating menopause and beyond, when energy levels fluctuate and motivation dips, this movement style can be the lifeline that keeps you moving through it all.

Ways to Exercise Snack

Category	Exercise Snack	Duration	Equipment Needed	Benefits
Strength	10 bodyweight squats	1 min	None	Leg strength, bone health
	5 push-ups (against wall or on knees)	1 min	None	Upper body and core strength
	10 chair sit-to-stands	2 mins	Chair	Glute and thigh activation
	30-second wall sit	30 secs	Wall	Quad and core endurance
Cardio	30-second fast marching on spot	30 secs	None	Heart health, circulation boost
	1-minute stair climbing	1 min	Stairs	Heart health, circulation boost
	2-minute dance burst to a favourite song	2 mins	Music	Joyful movement, mental lift

Mobility/ Flexibility	3 cat cow stretches	1 min	Mat (optional)	Spine mobility, posture improvement
	5 hip circles standing	1 min	None	Hip joint mobility, lower back release
	Forward fold and shoulder rolls	1–2 mins	None	Stretching, tension release
Balance	Single leg stand (30 secs per side)	1 min	None	Ankle strength, proprioception
	Heel-to-toe walk across room	2 mins	None	Coordination, fall prevention
Core	Seated knee lifts (on chair)	1 min	Chair	Core activation
	Standing side bends (with/without light weights)	2 mins	Optional light weights	Waistline mobility, oblique strength

CHAPTER 8

Hormones, Ageing and Exercise

As women, we often don't realise how interconnected our bodies are until something begins to shift. Ageing doesn't just happen at the surface. It's happening quietly in our bones, muscles, joints, hearts and even in how we think and feel. At the heart of many of these changes is a simple but powerful force: our hormones.

Hormones are your body's messengers, influencing everything from metabolism and mood to sleep patterns, stress management, fat storage and even the functioning of your skin, bones and brain. During perimenopause and menopause, as oestrogen and progesterone start to decline, many women experience a wave of unpredictable symptoms, including weight gain, brain fog, low energy, poor sleep and emotional fluctuations.[32]

But the decline in oestrogen isn't just about hot flushes or sleepless nights. It's a biological shift that affects every system in our body, influencing how we age, how long we live and the quality of our lives.

Understanding this connection and learning how to support our bodies through exercise is one of the greatest gifts we can give ourselves for the decades ahead.

Bone health

Our bones feel solid and reliable for many years, and we rarely give them much thought. Yet by the time we reach menopause, something significant is happening to our bone density. It begins to decline at an accelerated rate, and we break it down faster than we can build it. Research shows that women can lose up to 20% of their bone mass in the first 5 to 7 years after menopause.[33] And that's not a minor loss; it's a shift that dramatically raises the risk of osteoporosis, a disease that weakens bones and leaves them fragile.

One of the most effective ways to slow this decline, alongside good movement and nutrition, is through hormone replacement therapy (HRT). Oestrogen plays a crucial role in maintaining bone density, and when levels drop after menopause, bones become more susceptible to fractures. Studies, including those by the National Institute for Health and Care Excellence (NICE) and the Women's Health Initiative (WHI), have shown that HRT significantly reduces the risk of osteoporotic fractures in postmenopausal women, particularly when started around the time of menopause.[34] While HRT isn't suitable for everyone, for many women it can be a powerful tool for protecting bone health when used as part of a broader approach that includes strength training, calcium and vitamin D.

Why does this matter for longevity?

Because a fracture, especially a hip fracture, can change the course of life instantly. Statistics reveal that one in two women over 50 will suffer a fracture related to osteoporosis, and among those who break a hip, up to 20% will die within a year.

When bones are strong, they anchor us to our independence. When they're weak, a simple fall can lead to hospitalisation, immobility and a rapid decline in overall health. Strength training; a diet rich in protein, calcium and vitamin D; and regular weight-bearing movement can help fortify the structures that keep us upright, mobile and independent.

Marian had always considered herself naturally active. She gardened, walked with friends and was constantly on the move, looking after her grandchildren. But strength training? She dismissed it as something for athletes or gym lovers, not her.

Then Marian slipped on a damp kitchen tile one winter morning and fell. It seemed minor at first, but an X-ray revealed a hip fracture. She was stunned. I thought I was too active for that sort of thing, she told me later, but my bones just weren't strong enough to catch me.

Her recovery was long. She lost muscle mass during her hospital stay. Her independence was suddenly in question. The confidence she'd always carried so effortlessly began to crack. The scariest part? No one had warned her that this was a real risk for women her age, especially postmenopause.

During her rehab, we began strength work slowly: resistance bands, light weights and functional movements that mimicked everyday actions. At first, it wasn't about fitness; it was about rebuilding trust in her body.

Marian is now 69 and an active member of the OYM community. She trains twice a week with weights, walks daily and proudly tells anyone who listens about the importance of future-proofing your frame. She says, 'I might never have broken that hip if I'd started this in my fifties. But at least now, I know I won't break the next one.'

Marian's story is a powerful reminder that longevity isn't just about living but about staying strong enough to live fully, on your terms.

Joint health

Joints are the hinges and pivots that allow us to move freely, but they, too, are affected by declining hormone levels. As oestrogen levels fall, the cartilage that cushions our joints can become thinner and less resilient, leading to stiffness, discomfort and, in some cases, arthritis.

If we don't protect our joint health, movement can start to feel harder, and when movement decreases, so does overall vitality. Studies have shown that individuals with limited mobility have a 30–50% higher risk of early death than those who remain active.[35]

Movement isn't just exercise; it's life itself. And it doesn't have to be extreme. Gentle strength training, walking and stretching help build resilience in joints, keeping you supple. Every time you move, you nourish your joints with blood flow and lubrication. Every step reminds your body that it is still vibrant and capable.

Muscle health

Muscle mass is often associated with aesthetics, such as toned arms and strong legs, but it's far more than that. Muscles protect against frailty, serve as your support system against falls and act as your engine for energy and metabolism.

After the age of 30, we lose around 3–5% of our muscle mass every decade, and menopause accelerates this process. The decline in key hormones, particularly oestrogen, testosterone and growth hormones, directly impacts our ability to maintain and build muscle. Without intervention, by the time we reach our seventies or eighties, we could have lost nearly half of the muscle we had in our youth.

Sarcopenia, the term for age-related muscle loss, isn't just a cosmetic concern. It's directly linked to increased mortality. Research shows that individuals with greater muscle mass have a 63% lower risk of early death.[36]

But here's the empowering truth: muscle is highly adaptable at any age. Strength training signals to your body to preserve and rebuild muscle tissue, especially with adequate protein intake. In practical terms, that means being able to carry shopping bags, climb stairs, rise from a chair and get to the loo without help – the basic movements that add up to a life lived fully and without dependency.

Heart health

Cardiovascular disease remains one of the leading causes of death worldwide, and after age 50, the risk of heart-related conditions increases significantly.[37] This happens because oestrogen offers natural protection against cardiovascular disease by supporting healthy cholesterol levels and vascular flexibility. As oestrogen declines, the risk of arterial plaque build-up and heart attacks rises.

Regular exercise strengthens the heart, improves circulation and helps regulate blood pressure and cholesterol levels. It also reduces inflammation, a key contributor to many age-related diseases.

Just 150 minutes of moderate exercise each week, around 20 minutes a day, can lower the risk of heart disease by 30–40%. Even walking 4,000 steps a day has been shown to significantly reduce overall mortality risk, with each additional 500 steps reducing cardiovascular risk by 7%.[38]

Protecting your heart isn't about marathons. It's about the quiet, consistent rhythm of daily effort, the habit of choosing to move, nourish and strengthen.

Brain health

Cognitive shifts can be the most alarming of all the changes that may feel unsettling during midlife. Forgetfulness, lost words and brain fog are real, and they are closely linked to the hormonal shifts that come with menopause.

Dr Lisa Mosconi, a neuroscientist and director of the Women's Brain Initiative at Weill Cornell Medicine, has been a leading voice in uncovering how menopause affects the female brain. Her groundbreaking research shows that oestrogen acts directly on the brain, fuelling energy production and protecting neural connections. When oestrogen levels fall, so too can cognitive sharpness, making symptoms like brain fog not just real, but biologically explainable.

But movement, again, holds profound power. Exercise stimulates the release of BDNF (brain-derived neurotrophic factor), a protein that supports brain health, learning and memory. According to Alzheimer's Research UK, inactive adults have nearly twice the risk of developing dementia compared to those who stay active. By choosing to move, you not only strengthen your muscles and heart but also protect your memories, personality and ability to connect with the world and the people you love.

Metabolic health

Exercise also plays a vital role in maintaining metabolic health, helping to regulate blood sugar levels and reducing the risk of type 2 diabetes. As we age, insulin sensitivity can decrease, making it harder for the body to process glucose efficiently. However, regular movement helps improve insulin function, stabilise energy levels and reduce the risk of metabolic disorders. Additionally, exercise supports immune function, allowing the body to fight infections and illnesses more effectively.

Movement and mood

Finally, movement is a natural mood booster. Exercise triggers the release of endorphins, serotonin and dopamine, hormones that enhance mood, reduce stress and help combat anxiety and depression. It also improves sleep quality, which is crucial for overall health and recovery. Many people assume that fatigue is inevitable as they age. However, regular movement increases energy levels by enhancing mitochondrial function, which enables the body to generate and utilise energy more efficiently.

A Little Bit of Important Science When It Comes to Understanding the Importance of Muscle in Longevity

I want to highlight something that is pretty scientific BUT is important to understand, and for those who love a little science, I think you'll enjoy. It is relatively new research that has significant implications for our future health and further emphasises how crucial muscle is for women.

You might not know what mitochondria, cytokines and myokines are, but they play a huge role in how well we age, especially as women. These tiny powerhouses help give us energy, reduce inflammation and support recovery. We can boost how well they work through movement, exercise and rest.

By staying active and giving our bodies time to recover, we support these powerful allies behind the scenes helping us feel stronger, more energised and better equipped to handle whatever midlife brings.

Mitochondria: the energy powerhouses keeping us young

These tiny structures inside our cells generate energy. They are often referred to as the powerhouse of the cell. However, as we age, our mitochondria start to decline. They become less efficient, meaning less energy for our cells and a higher likelihood of fatigue, metabolic slowdowns and even chronic diseases. This process is called mitochondrial dysfunction, a key driver of ageing.

How can we maintain our mitochondria's functionality as they were in our twenties? Exercise. Movement stimulates the process of making more mitochondria, and resistance training, cardio and high-intensity interval training (HIIT) have been shown to upregulate this process.[39] More mitochondria mean better energy production, improved metabolism and a slower ageing body.

Cytokines: inflammation or not

These small proteins help regulate inflammation and immune responses in the body. Some cytokines are beneficial and promote healing, while others contribute to chronic inflammation, which is linked to everything from heart disease to osteoporosis to cognitive decline. This can be confusing because ageing is associated with a rise in these pro-inflammatory cytokines.

Once again, exercise and movement are the most effective methods for controlling cytokines. Moderate physical activity reduces chronic low-grade inflammation by promoting anti-inflammatory cytokines, while suppressing harmful ones. Strength training, yoga and walking all contribute to a balanced cytokine environment, helping to maintain a strong immune system and a resilient body.

Myokines

Myokines, released by our muscles during exercise, play a massive role in longevity. They are like the body's internal medicine, helping reduce inflammation, improve metabolism, enhance insulin sensitivity and support brain health. One of the most powerful myokines, irisin, has been shown to stimulate fat-burning, protect against neurodegeneration and support cardiovascular health.

Strength training is particularly effective in boosting myokine production. When we lift weights or engage in resistance training, our muscles send signals promoting cellular repair and longevity. This is why strength training is non-negotiable for women as we age. Strong muscles don't just make us look and feel good; they communicate with the rest of our body to keep us functioning optimally for decades.

Before you assume that longevity requires constant workouts, it doesn't. Rest and recovery are equally essential. Overtraining or ignoring recovery can backfire, raising stress hormones and inflammation, which disrupts mitochondrial function and cytokine balance.

It is crucial to prioritise quality sleep, active recovery (such as yoga or walking) and stress management techniques (like journalling), which we will focus on in this book and the accompanying plan. Our body does most of its repair work while we sleep, clearing out damaged cells, reducing inflammation and optimising mitochondrial function. If you're skimping on rest, even the best exercise routine won't work.

PART 2.2
Nutrition

During perimenopause and menopause, declining oestrogen levels lead to a natural shift in how our bodies function. As established in the previous chapter, we lose muscle mass more easily, metabolism slows and changes in fat distribution, mood and energy become apparent. This is why nutrition is more important than ever. A diet rich in whole foods can enhance hormone balance, protect your bones, support your brain and boost your energy. Conversely, poor nutrition can leave you feeling flat, foggy, inflamed and frustrated.

CHAPTER 9

Fuelling Your Body for Longevity

One of the most powerful lessons I've learnt from my own experiences and from supporting thousands of women through midlife is that what we eat influences how we age. This goes beyond our waistlines or weight; it affects how we feel, think and sleep and how well our bodies function as the years go by.

As our hormones begin to shift during perimenopause and menopause, many women feel as though their bodies are working against them. Energy slumps, disrupted sleep, increased anxiety, brain fog and stubborn weight gain are not merely signs of ageing; they indicate that the inner systems that once operated on autopilot now require additional support. This support can begin with our diet.

Nutrition is one of the most powerful tools we have for feeling better today and building resilience for the future. The meals you eat can influence everything from mood and metabolism to bone strength, immune function and even how sharp your mind stays later in life.

That's why the meals in this plan are built around foods that nourish you from the inside out, particularly plants, because they offer so much of what your body needs in this phase of life. But this isn't about cutting things out or sticking to rules. It's about learning how to fuel your body wisely and kindly, with real, enjoyable food that supports the woman you are now and the woman you want to be in 10, 20 or 30 years.

There is so much confusion over what balance means and what a nourishing meal looks like, so let's break it down.

Macronutrients

Your body needs macronutrients, such as carbohydrates, proteins, healthy fats and fibre that support various functions. Together, these elements fuel your cells, regulate hormones, protect your brain and help prevent chronic diseases.

Carbohydrates: energy, hormone support and longevity

Carbs have had a bad rap in recent years, especially in the wellness space. But the truth is, carbohydrates are your body's primary source of energy, and they play a crucial role in hormone health and longevity.

When chosen well, carbs help stabilise blood sugar, fuel your brain, support thyroid function and feed the good bacteria in your gut. They also help regulate cortisol, the stress hormone, and reduce cravings by keeping you satisfied.

The key is to focus on complex, fibre-rich carbohydrates found in whole, unprocessed foods like:

- sweet potatoes
- brown rice

- quinoa
- oats
- lentils, beans and chickpeas
- vegetables like squash, beetroot and carrots
- fruits like berries, apples and citrus
- wholegrain breads and pastas

Around 40–50% of your total daily intake should come from quality carbohydrates. That means including some in each main meal – enough to feel satisfied, energised and stable throughout the day, without the crash.[40]

Protein: the midlife powerhouse nutrient

Protein becomes even more essential as we age, especially for women transitioning through menopause. Declining oestrogen leads to muscle and bone loss, slower recovery and changes in metabolism. Protein helps slow this process, rebuilds tissue, supports hormone production and preserves strength.

It also regulates appetite by keeping you feeling fuller for longer and aiding in blood sugar control. Many women aren't consuming enough protein, particularly if they are busy, stressed or skipping meals.

Aim for 1–1.2 grams of protein per kilogram of body weight each day. For a 70kg woman, that's approximately 70–84 grams daily, ideally distributed across your meals. Your body cannot absorb large amounts at once, so consistent intake is essential.

Here's what a protein-rich day might look like:

- **Breakfast**: Greek yoghurt with chia seeds and berries (20g)

- **Lunch**: Quinoa and lentil salad with roasted veg and tahini (25g)

- **Dinner**: Grilled salmon with leafy greens and sweet potato (30g)

- **Snack (if needed)**: Hummus with oatcakes, boiled egg or a small protein smoothie (10–15g)

If you notice that you're tired soon after meals, are snacking more at night or experiencing cravings or low energy late in the day, it could be a sign that you're not getting enough protein. For some, adding a mid-afternoon protein snack can help avoid the common pattern of mindless evening eating.

Healthy fats

Healthy fats are essential, not just tolerated but necessary for hormone production, brain health and mood regulation. They reduce inflammation, support skin and joint health and help the body absorb key fat-soluble vitamins, including A, D, E and K.

Excellent sources of healthy fat include:

- avocados

- extra virgin olive oil

- nuts and seeds

- oily fish (like salmon and sardines)

- nut butters and tahini

Fibre

Fibre is just as crucial. It promotes regular digestion, nourishes gut bacteria, supports oestrogen detoxification and helps reduce the risk of heart disease, diabetes and hormone-driven cancers. You should be aiming for 30g a day. You'll find it in:

- legumes (lentils, beans and chickpeas)
- vegetables and fruits (especially with skins and seeds)
- whole grains (quinoa, oats, brown rice)
- nuts and seeds

Aiming for 30 different plant foods per week can work wonders for gut and hormone health.

And don't forget hydration; water is essential for digestion, circulation and detoxification. Aim for 1.5–2 litres per day.

Micronutrients

Alongside macronutrients, you also need a steady supply of key vitamins and minerals to feel and function your best:

- **Vitamin D:** Supports bone density and immune function.
- **Magnesium:** Eases anxiety, improves sleep and supports muscle relaxation.
- **Iron:** Helps prevent fatigue and brain fog, especially during the post-menstrual years.
- **Vitamin B complex:** Important for mood, energy and nervous system health.

- **Omega-3s:** Help regulate inflammation, support brain function and ease joint pain.

Deficiencies in any of these, especially if you're under stress or not eating well, can contribute to anxiety, fatigue, depression and poor concentration.

A nutrient-rich, balanced diet isn't about restriction or clean eating. It's about making sustainable, supportive choices that help your body age well, feel good and stay strong.

You don't have to track every bite or follow a complicated food plan. Instead, focus on building balanced meals, staying hydrated and consistently choosing whole, nourishing foods. Small shifts, such as adding protein to your breakfast, swapping white carbs for whole grains or incorporating healthy fats into each meal, can create significant changes in how you feel and function.

Macronutrients and where to find them

Macronutrient	Function in the Body	Food Sources
Protein	Builds and repairs tissues, supports immune function, makes enzymes and hormones.	Chicken, turkey, fish, eggs, Greek yogurt, tofu, lentils, chickpeas, tempeh, quinoa, cottage cheese
Carbohydrates	Primary energy source for the brain and muscles during exercise.	Whole grains (brown rice, oats, quinoa), fruits, vegetables, legumes, sweet potatoes
Fats	Supports cell growth, protects organs, helps absorb nutrients and produces hormones.	Avocados, nuts, seeds, olive oil, oily fish (salmon, sardines), flaxseeds, chia seeds
Fibre (carb)	Supports digestion, helps maintain blood sugar levels, aids in satiety.	Whole grains, vegetables, fruits (especially with skins), legumes, flaxseeds, chia seeds
Water	Regulates body temperature, transports nutrients, removes waste, essential for all functions.	Water, herbal teas, fruits and vegetables (like cucumber, watermelon, celery)

Why Plants Hold the Key to a Longer Life

If there's one thing we know about the people who thrive into their nineties and beyond, it's this: they primarily eat plants. And that's not a coincidence. A plant-based diet consistently stands out when it comes to future-proofing your body, boosting energy, reducing disease risk and maintaining active and independent well-being well into later life.

It's not about being perfect or rigid; it's about choosing foods that support your body, brain and hormones with every bite. And that's precisely why most of the meals in this plan are plant-based. Plants are nutritional powerhouses, packed with fibre, antioxidants, vitamins, minerals and anti-inflammatory compounds that shield your cells from ageing and disease.

- Fibre keeps your gut microbiome healthy, which plays a significant role in everything from mood to immunity and hormone balance.
- Antioxidants in colourful vegetables and fruits combat the daily damage caused by stress, pollution and even exercise.
- Plant compounds such as polyphenols found in berries, olive oil, spices and herbs help reduce inflammation, enhance brain health and support heart function.

When we primarily consume plants, we naturally eliminate ultra-processed foods, excess sugar and unhealthy fats, which accelerate ageing, disrupt our moods and deplete our energy.

Less Meat, More Life

Let's discuss meat.

Or rather, let's consider why reducing your consumption of it may be one of the wisest choices for your long-term health.

Before you panic, I'm not here to tell you to cut it all out. I haven't.

I eat fish and white meat because I love the nourishment they provide. The key for me, and what I've integrated into this plan, is balance, not restriction or extremes. It's simply about enjoying more of the good foods, more often.

Multiple studies have linked high consumption of red and processed meats to increased health risks:

- **Cardiovascular disease:** A comprehensive review by the University of Oxford found that a higher intake of red and processed meats is associated with an elevated risk of heart disease.[41]

- **Type 2 diabetes:** Research from the Harvard T.H. Chan School of Public Health indicates that individuals consuming the most red meat had a 62% higher risk of developing Type 2 diabetes compared to those consuming the least. Each additional daily serving of processed red meat was linked to a 46% greater risk.[42]

- **Cancer:** The World Health Organization classifies processed meats as Group 1 carcinogens, meaning there is sufficient evidence that they cause cancer, particularly colorectal cancer.[43]

These findings underpin the importance of moderating red and processed meat intake to reduce the risk of chronic diseases.

It's not about cutting out red meat entirely though, it's about becoming more conscious of quality, portion and frequency, and pairing it with whole, colourful foods that bring balance. When meat is eaten alongside plenty of fibre-rich vegetables, whole grains and healthy fats, it has a very different impact within the body. The fibre helps regulate digestion and supports a healthy gut microbiome, both of which play a critical role in hormone metabolism.

Your gut and liver are key players in breaking down and clearing out excess hormones, especially oestrogen. If either is under strain due to poor diet, alcohol, stress or lack of sleep, it can lead to imbalances that show up as mood swings, PMS-like symptoms, hot flushes or stubborn weight gain.

You don't have to overhaul everything. Small shifts, such as swapping processed meats for plant-forward meals a few times a week or opting for slow-cooked, grass-fed options instead of chargrilled or fried, can reduce the inflammatory load and support your body's natural rhythms.

A great deal of what I've learnt while writing this book comes from studying the habits of people who live the longest, healthiest lives, particularly those in the Blue Zones. Despite their geographical and cultural differences, they share one standout trait: their diets are predominantly plant-based.

In regions such as Okinawa, Ikaria, Sardinia, the Nicoya Peninsula and Loma Linda (home to a large community of Seventh-Day Adventists), up to 95% of the diet consists of whole plant foods. Beans play a starring role, whether it's black beans in Costa Rica, soybeans in Okinawa or lentils and chickpeas in the Mediterranean zones. These staples are rich in protein, fibre and slow-releasing carbohydrates, offering sustained energy and supporting smooth digestion.

In these communities, meat isn't off limits, but it's eaten sparingly, typically just a few times a month and often as part of cultural or family traditions. In Loma Linda, where many follow vegetarian or pescatarian lifestyles, people live 7–10 years longer than the US average, and chronic disease rates are dramatically lower.[44]

I haven't eaten red meat in over 35 years. I choose to eat fish and some white meat, and I centre most of my meals around plants. This isn't about perfection, it's about balance and longevity. The Blue Zones demonstrate that it's not extreme measures or restrictive diets that support long-term health, but rather simple, consistent habits that nourish the body over time. These individuals aren't chasing the latest wellness trends or obsessing over every bite. They're living in a way that naturally supports vitality, and the results speak for themselves.

CHAPTER 10

Hormones, Ageing and Nutrition

Midlife is a time of change in our roles, responsibilities, mindsets and bodies. One of the most significant changes occurring behind the scenes is the natural shift in hormones. While we can't stop this process, we can powerfully support it through the way we nourish ourselves.

Here's the truth I want every woman to know about ageing: you're not powerless, and you don't have to just put up with it. The right nutrition can help rebalance your body, and lay the groundwork for better long-term health.

One of the lesser-known disruptors of hormonal health is blood sugar instability. When we eat foods that spike our blood sugar – such as refined carbs, sugary snacks or meals low in protein and fibre – our body responds by releasing insulin. After the spike comes the crash, which triggers cortisol, our primary stress hormone.

Chronically high cortisol levels interfere with sleep, increase fat storage (particularly around the middle) and can worsen mood swings and anxiety.

That's why building every meal with a balance of protein, fibre and healthy fats is so effective. This combination helps to stabilise your blood sugar, calm cortisol and reduce those highs and lows that leave you feeling drained and irritable. Over time, this one shift can have a dramatic impact on energy, sleep, cravings and mood.

As we age, low-grade chronic inflammation also becomes more prevalent, especially when hormone levels fluctuate.[45] This type of inflammation often manifests as joint pain, skin flare-ups, digestive issues and brain fog. If left unchecked, it can elevate the risk of heart disease, diabetes and cognitive decline.

But food can be part of the solution.

Anti-inflammatory foods like colourful vegetables, leafy greens, oily fish, extra virgin olive oil, nuts, seeds, turmeric and berries are rich in antioxidants and omega-3 fatty acids. They actively help calm inflammation in the body, improve mental clarity, and even enhance mood.

In my early forties, I began noticing subtle shifts. At first, it was little things: mid-afternoon slumps, restless sleep and cravings that hit hard after lunch. I felt like I was running on empty more often, and reaching for sugary snacks became a quick fix I relied on.

I told myself I was just tired and busy, but deep down, I knew I needed to make a change.

So, I started paying closer attention to my meals. I added more protein to breakfast, swapped out the processed snacks for nuts, fruit and seeds, and began prioritising omega-3s through oily fish and flaxseeds. These small tweaks had a huge impact. I felt calmer, less bloated, more balanced and much more in control of my energy and appetite. It wasn't about being perfect; it was about being intentional in noticing what my body needed and consistently providing it with care.

I've seen the same results with so many of the women I've worked with. Everything changes when we stop focusing on eating less and start focusing on eating better. You begin to feel like yourself again: more grounded, energised, clear-headed and strong.

As hormone levels drop, our metabolism slows, and fat storage shifts, particularly to the abdominal area. It's not just frustrating; it increases the risk of type 2 diabetes, cardiovascular disease and hormone-sensitive cancers. Oestrogen also helps protect bone density and cognitive function, so when it declines, our risk of osteoporosis and memory issues increases, too.

By focusing on nutrient-dense, anti-inflammatory whole foods and minimising ultra-processed ones, you're supporting your bones, heart, brain and emotional well-being for the long run.

This isn't about restriction or chasing perfection; it's about making sustainable, nourishing choices – small shifts that accumulate over time. Opt for whole grains instead of refined ones, add protein to your breakfast, replace crisps or biscuits with seeds, eggs or yoghurt, and drink more water. Include something green on your plate each day.

When you eat with intention, you stabilise your hormones, support your gut, reduce inflammation and give your body the building blocks it needs to age well.

CHAPTER 11

What to Eat to Support Your Mind and Slow Age-Related Cognitive Decline

What we eat doesn't just affect our bodies – it deeply shapes our minds, too. While much of the conversation around ageing tends to focus on physical changes like muscle loss, joint stiffness or weight gain, the brain is quietly undergoing its own transformation. The good news is that we can support our cognitive health and emotional resilience through the food we eat every day.

As we age, the brain becomes increasingly vulnerable to oxidative stress, inflammation and imbalances in blood sugar. If left unchecked, these factors can impair concentration, memory and mood and even heighten the risk of cognitive diseases such as Alzheimer's. However, nutrition provides us with a powerful tool to help slow this process. The goal isn't merely to live longer, it's to remain sharp, connected and mentally vibrant for as long as possible.

Nutrients for brain protection

Certain nutrients play a key role in protecting the brain. Omega-3 fatty acids, found in oily fish like salmon and sardines, as well as flaxseeds, chia seeds and walnuts, are essential for building and maintaining healthy brain cells. They also help reduce inflammation in the brain, supporting better mood, clearer thinking and memory retention. B vitamins, especially B6, B12 and folate, are vital for brain energy and nerve function. Low levels of these vitamins have been linked with poor memory, brain fog and even higher risks of dementia. Leafy greens, eggs, beans and whole grains are wonderful sources.

Antioxidants and polyphenols for protection from cellular damage

Then there are antioxidants and polyphenols, the unsung heroes that protect your brain from cellular damage. These powerful compounds combat oxidative stress, a major driver of ageing. Foods such as blueberries, raspberries, dark chocolate, green tea and extra virgin olive oil are rich in these protective nutrients and can significantly impact cognitive longevity. Minerals like magnesium and zinc are also essential for calming the nervous system and supporting a stable mood. They are found in foods like pumpkin seeds, legumes and spinach and are especially important when stress or disrupted sleep begins to affect how you feel and think. Vitamin D, which is often low in the UK, also plays a crucial role, not only for bone and immune health but also for reducing neurological inflammation and maintaining mood balance.

An anti-inflammatory diet

Another factor quietly affecting cognitive ageing is chronic, low-grade inflammation. This kind of background stress contributes to joint stiffness, fatigue and mental sluggishness. Left unchecked, it's also linked to depression and degenerative brain diseases. This is why an anti-inflammatory diet can be such a game-changer. Brightly coloured vegetables, leafy greens, oily fish, berries, olive oil, nuts, seeds, turmeric and ginger all help calm inflammation and protect the brain. Reducing foods that drive inflammation, like refined sugars, processed snacks, excess alcohol and trans fats, is just as important. It's not about cutting everything out but about consistently choosing foods that nourish, not drain, your energy.

Supporting hormonal balance

Hormonal shifts during perimenopause and menopause don't just impact the body; they also affect the brain. It's why so many women report changes in memory, focus and mood during this phase of life. Oestrogen plays a role in cognitive function, and when it declines, it can trigger brain fog, irritability and a general feeling of being 'off'. Supporting hormonal balance through a balanced diet can have a powerful knock-on effect on your mental and emotional well-being. Flaxseeds, pumpkin seeds, cruciferous vegetables like broccoli and kale, magnesium-rich foods like spinach and almonds, and fermented foods help support hormone clearance, reduce stress and improve sleep and mood.

Hydration

Hydration is another quiet but essential factor. The brain is composed of nearly 75% water, and even mild dehydration can impair memory, cause headaches and impact mood. Drinking around 2 litres of water a day alongside herbal teas, hydrating foods like cucumber and melon, and a little coconut water for electrolytes can make a big difference in how clear and focused you feel.

By fuelling your brain with whole, nutrient-dense, anti-inflammatory foods and staying hydrated, you give yourself the best chance to think, feel emotionally steady and remain mentally engaged at every stage of life. It's not about being perfect, it's about consistency. A few nourishing habits practised daily can completely change the way you age.

CHAPTER 12

The Gut Feeling

If there's one thing that links your energy, mood, immunity, weight and even how well you age, it's your gut.

We often think of the gut as just a digestive machine, but it's the command centre for your entire health ecosystem. It's where 70% of your immune system lives and is home to trillions of bacteria that digest food and help regulate hormones, control inflammation and communicate directly with your brain via the gut–brain axis.[46] This makes it a cornerstone of longevity and deeply connected to movement, nutrition and mental well-being, the pillars we're building sustainable habits around.

Why a Healthy Gut Matters More in Midlife

In midlife and beyond, hormonal shifts can increase gut sensitivity and reduce microbial diversity. That's science-speak for: you may feel bloated more often, notice changes in your bowel habits, experience food sensitivities or feel more anxious than usual. A well-fed, balanced gut can ease these transitions and even help you better absorb nutrients vital for bone health, muscle recovery and cognitive clarity.

This is where a plant-predominant diet becomes your superpower.

Think of your gut like a garden. The more diverse the plants, the more thriving and resilient they become. Each type of fibre from vegetables, fruits, legumes, nuts, seeds and whole grains feeds different beneficial bacteria. This diversity helps create a more balanced microbiome, which has been shown to:

- lower inflammation (a key driver of chronic disease and ageing)
- improve insulin sensitivity
- regulate weight
- enhance mood and mental resilience

Crucially, plant-based diets are rich in prebiotics (the food for good bacteria) and polyphenols, which support the growth of bacteria that produce short-chain fatty acids like butyrate, which are known for protecting the gut lining and reducing inflammation.

You don't need to be fully plant-based to see benefits. Even shifting towards 30 different plant foods per week has been shown to boost gut diversity.[47]

Mental Well-Being: The Gut-Brain Connection for Longevity

You've probably felt those butterflies in your stomach before a big moment or a wave of nausea when you're stressed. That's not your imagination. That's your gut talking to your brain.

The gut–brain axis is a powerful two-way communication highway. When your gut is inflamed or imbalanced, it sends distress signals that ripple through your body, raising anxiety, lowering mood, disrupting sleep and ultimately chipping away at your long-term health. This becomes especially important during perimenopause and menopause, when our natural serotonin levels start to dip, and stress can feel more intense than ever.

Why does this matter for longevity? The state of your gut doesn't just influence how you feel today; it plays a critical role in how you'll feel years from now. A well-functioning gut supports your immune system, helps regulate hormones, balances inflammation and even protects brain function, all vital for ageing well.

Your gut microbiome, home to trillions of bacteria, is central to this process. A healthy, diverse microbiome helps synthesise key neurotransmitters like serotonin and GABA, which help us feel calm, clear-headed and emotionally steady. It's no exaggeration to say that your gut is a cornerstone of your mental and emotional resilience.

I remember working with Jenny, who came to me feeling overwhelmed. She had bloating, anxiety and was barely sleeping. She assumed it was just part of menopause. But we took it step by step. We added in fermented foods like sauerkraut and kefir, boosted her fibre with plant diversity, and introduced regular walks and simple moments of connection. Within weeks, the bloating eased. Her sleep deepened. And, most importantly, she felt like herself again. Calm, capable and in control.

It perfectly shows how supporting gut health isn't about deprivation. It's about gentle, powerful additions that support your vitality now and long into the future.

Let's be clear: it's not just what you eat, it's how you live.

Movement is a gut health hero. Regular physical activity increases gut motility, keeping your digestion smooth and efficient, and boosts microbial diversity, which strengthens your gut lining and supports your metabolism. Whether it's a walk after dinner, some resistance training or a mobility session, every bit of movement contributes to a healthier gut and a more vibrant, longer life.

Remember, gut health is not about cutting out everything that brings you joy. It's about layering in habits that support how you want to feel today *and* how you want to age. Small changes, repeated consistently, create the conditions for long-term resilience.

Here's a great place to start:

- Aim for 30 different plants each week (diversity is key).
- Include legumes for fibre and resistant starch.
- Eat root vegetables and leafy greens (rich in prebiotics).
- Enjoy berries and herbs (high in polyphenols).
- Try fermented foods like kefir, sauerkraut and kimchi.
- Hydrate well – your gut lining depends on it.

And don't underestimate the power of emotional nourishment. Chronic stress alters the microbiome and suppresses digestion. Your nervous system and gut thrive when you carve out space for calm. Whether it's a walk in nature, breathwork, time with loved ones or simply laughter, these moments of joy and stillness are just as critical as what's on your plate.

Your gut is a foundation for your future. Support it well, and it will support you through menopause, into older age, and for the long life you're building with purpose.

Longevity Lens: A Happy Gut, a Longer Life

Research has linked gut diversity to healthy ageing, reduced frailty and lower all-cause mortality.[48] When your gut is balanced, your whole body functions better, your immune system is sharper, your hormones are steadier, and your mental health is more resilient.

There are many ways we can help support our gut microbiome. By making minor, sustainable tweaks, you will begin to feel the benefits and may start to see an improvement in your gut health.

This table shows you ways to add an array of essential foods to boost your gut health and support the good bacteria.

Ways to boost your gut health

ADD	WHAT	BENEFIT
FIBRE (Soluble)	Oats, fruits (figs, kiwis, pears, apples), carrots and beans	Great for maintaining healthy cholesterol and feeding our gut.
FIBRE (Insoluble)	Whole grains, nuts, seeds, cauliflower and legumes	Helps bulk up stools and increase motility in the gut.
PREBIOTICS	Onions, leeks, garlic, mushrooms, asparagus, green beans, chicory, beetroot, green bananas, nuts and grains	Feeds the good bacteria.
PROBIOTICS	Fermented foods, such as kefir, live yoghurt, miso, kimchi, sauerkraut and kombucha	Populates your gut with good bacteria.
PLANTS	Aim for 30 different-coloured plant foods per week, including all herbs, spices, nuts, seeds, fruits and veggies. Try broccoli, chia seeds, lentils, beans, asparagus, avocado, seeds, beetroot, apples, sweet potato and red pepper	Plant-based foods contain lots of fibre as well as vitamins, minerals, antioxidants and phytonutrients, all of which we need in abundance as our bodies mature and hormones fluctuate. These foods will help protect against heart disease, obesity, high blood pressure, diabetes and some cancers. Plant-based foods will support your hormone balance, immunity and mood.

Incorporating gut-nourishing habits during your 21-Day Plan will give you a strong foundation for feeling better now and ageing with vitality and independence.

On pages 296–312 you will find five of my favourite, mostly plant-based breakfasts, lunches and dinners that contain everything you need to ensure you hit the targets. I hope these dishes also prove that we don't need to overcomplicate our choices and that you can build sensible and achievable habits around food with lots of preparation and commitment.

CHAPTER 13

How to Eat: Mindful Eating and Intermittent Fasting

When we think about ageing well, the first thing that usually comes to mind is what we're eating: more colourful vegetables, less sugar, more protein and more fibre. But here's the thing: how you eat can be just as important. I know it sounds simple, but the way you approach your meals – how fast you eat, how much attention you give your food, and even when you choose to eat – can have a massive impact on everything from your metabolism to your hormones, gut health, mood and future health.

Let's break it down and discuss two concepts: enter mindful eating and intermittent fasting. They are entirely different, and neither has to be perfect or complicated, but both can significantly enhance your health, especially during midlife.

Mindful Eating: Tuning Back In

Mindful eating is exactly what it sounds like: eating with awareness. It involves slowing down, properly tasting your food and genuinely checking in to see how hungry or full you feel. It's about pressing pause on autopilot eating (you know, when you're halfway through a snack and suddenly realise you weren't even hungry) and giving your meals your full attention.

It's about reconnecting with what your body is asking for and allowing yourself to listen. I used to eat on the go, but now I make an effort to sit and savour my food. This way, you can honour your fullness, and it prevents you from picking and grazing, which can disrupt the microbiome and may cause you to eat more than you need.

Why mindful eating matters for women, especially in midlife:
- **It aids digestion:** Eating slowly allows your body to produce the enzymes and stomach acid necessary for properly breaking down food, reducing the likelihood of feeling bloated or sluggish afterwards.
- **It balances blood sugar:** Being more aware of what and how you eat can help prevent the blood sugar rollercoaster that leaves you feeling tired, cranky and constantly reaching for snacks.
- **It reduces inflammation:** Stress eating, eating on the go or scoffing food while distracted can trigger low-grade inflammation in the body, which we now know plays a big role in how we age.
- **It regulates hunger hormones:** If you're eating too fast, your body doesn't have time to register fullness. That's when those tricky hormones (leptin and ghrelin) go out of whack, often leading to overeating.
- **It supports your mental well-being:** Mindful eating can break the cycle of emotional eating, a huge one for women

dealing with mood swings, anxiety or stress during the menopause years.

Simple things like putting your fork down between bites, eating without your phone or even taking a few breaths before you start eating can change how your body responds to food. Over time, these little habits help reduce that 'tired but wired' feeling, support your gut and make you feel more in control of your eating without going anywhere near restriction.

Intermittent Fasting: Giving Your Body a Break

Now, let's talk about something that's been buzzing around lately: intermittent fasting or, as I like to call it, time-based eating! It's not about restricting calories or sticking to a rigid plan. Instead, it's all about simply narrowing the window during which you enjoy your meals, like having your meals between 10 a.m. and 6 p.m.

Sounds simple, and giving your body a proper break from digestion can do a lot of good.

Here's what the research (and experience) tells us intermittent fasting can support:[49]

- **Better metabolism:** Fasting helps your body transition from burning sugar for energy to burning fat, which supports insulin sensitivity – a significant factor for women in midlife.

- **Reduced inflammation:** Digesting food around the clock puts a load on your body. Fasting gives your gut and immune system a breather.

- **Cellular clean-up:** Fasting triggers an amazing process called autophagy. It's as if your cells are conducting a thorough spring clean, eliminating the old or damaged ones and making space for the new.

- **Weight regulation:** Eating within a shorter window naturally reduces the chances of overeating or snacking late into the night without needing to count a single calorie.

- **Better gut health:** Giving your digestive system time off supports a more balanced microbiome, which means happier hormones, more energy and even better sleep.

I practised intermittent fasting because it suited my rhythm, but something changed. Now, I usually stop eating around 7 p.m. and have what is now known as a 'proffee' – protein coffee offering 30g of protein – first thing the next morning to fuel my workout. I then refuel after my workout at around 9:30 a.m. This routine helps me feel clear-headed and energised, and it has become a staple in my life without ever feeling restrictive.

This is key; I don't force it. I eat if I've had a rough night's sleep, feel off or know I need something earlier. There is no guilt, no rules. It's about working with my body, not against it.

When I break my fast, I ensure that I do so with a protein-rich meal to support my muscles, hormones and blood sugar. That first meal sets the tone for the day, especially in midlife when energy, focus and mood can fluctuate.

But is it right for you?

This is where it becomes intriguing. Intermittent fasting has been extensively researched in men and younger individuals, but women in midlife present a unique case. Our hormones are more sensitive to stress, and fasting, especially if done too aggressively or without adequate nourishment, can be a stressor.

So, it's about tuning in (just like with mindful eating) and watching how your body responds.

Fasting might not be working for you if you notice:

- you're more anxious or irritable
- your sleep is disrupted
- your energy is dwindling or you feel foggy
- your cycle becomes irregular or your hormones feel out of whack

If that's the case, it's perfectly fine to scale back. A gentle 12-hour overnight fast is still extremely beneficial and much more supportive for many women than forcing themselves to endure something that simply doesn't feel right.

Ultimately, both mindful eating and intermittent fasting emphasise establishing a rhythm that allows for a nourishing, supportive and sustainable approach to eating. It's not something to master overnight or dwell on excessively. Instead, it represents a gradual return to tuning into your body and providing it with the space and attention it truly deserves.

When you start eating this way – more consciously, more in sync with your body – you might be surprised how much easier it is to feel energised, grounded and, yes, even youthful.

Because longevity isn't about chasing perfection, it's about building habits that help you feel better now and keep you strong, calm and capable in the long run.

CHAPTER 14

Do Supplements Support?

While nutrition should always be the primary focus in supporting longevity, supplements can play a valid and beneficial role, provided a strong dietary foundation has been established. Whole foods provide a rich, complex array of nutrients, fibre and phytochemicals that work together to support everything from hormone balance to brain function. A diet centred on plants, healthy fats, quality proteins and minimal ultra-processed foods lays the groundwork for longevity by reducing inflammation, stabilising blood sugar, protecting gut health and supporting muscle and bone integrity.

However, as we age, especially through midlife and beyond, there are times when even the most nutritious diet may fall short, whether due to lifestyle demands, reduced absorption, changes in appetite, or increased physiological needs. This is where carefully selected supplements can offer meaningful support. They're not a replacement for good nutrition but can help bridge the gaps, reinforce key systems and optimise long-term health.

The key is to view supplements as targeted tools, not blanket solutions. Many people reach for them without understanding what their bodies need, resulting in unnecessary expense or imbalance. When chosen mindfully, and ideally guided by testing or professional input, supplements can complement the efforts you're already making through food, movement, sleep and stress management.

The table below outlines some of the most beneficial supplements for midlife and longevity, explaining why they matter, who might benefit most and what to look for when choosing them.

Key nutrients and where to find them[50]

Nutrient	Where can I find it?	Why do I need it?
Vitamin C (ascorbic acid)	Red peppers, oranges, kiwis, mangoes, berries, tomatoes, broccoli, green leafy vegetables, parsley, blackcurrants and frozen peas are all good choices. Eat daily.	Vitamin C is a powerful antioxidant and is easy to consume. It improves the health of our cells, heart and immune system and can help during times of stress – a common symptom of perimenopause. It also helps to produce collagen, which is in decline at this stage of life.
Vitamin B6	Milk, salmon, tuna, eggs, chicken liver, beef, carrots, spinach, sweet potato, green peas, bananas, chickpeas, cereal and avocado. Incorporate these into your diet daily.	Curtails low mood, mood swings and depression by helping to produce a key chemical messenger, serotonin. During menopause, serotonin levels fluctuate or drop, which can also contribute to brain fog, dizziness, heart palpitations, vertigo and memory problems.
Vitamin B12	Most commonly found in animal products – fish, meat, poultry and eggs.	Key for boosting energy, brain health, memory, bone health and your overall mood and well-being. If you are a vegetarian and suffer from low energy, fatigue, memory loss, constipation, loss of appetite, numbness and tingling in the hands and feet or depression, it would be well worth getting your B12 levels tested by your GP.
Calcium	Dairy or fortified plant milk, tinned fish with bones (such as sardines and whitebait), tofu, spinach, broccoli, white beans, dried figs, almonds, oranges, kale and watercress. Under the age of 50, women need around 700mg of calcium daily, and after 50, this increases to 1200mg daily.	Calcium levels decrease with age, especially in women after menopause. It is essential for healthy bones, teeth, heart and muscles. Unless advised by your doctor, stay away from supplementing.

Vitamin D	Expose your skin to sunshine! Other sources include fatty fish, fish liver oils, beef liver, cheese, egg yolks, and fortified foods. Include as much as you can into your daily diet and get outside in the sunshine daily.	Vitamin D is important for bone health, helping prevent brittle bones and bone pain, and osteomalacia (softening of the bones). It is also important for a healthy immune system. Although it can be obtained from a few food sources, the sun is the best source. For this reason, it is a nutrient we often need to supplement, especially in the West and during the winter. Aim for D3 form, ideally coupled with K2, as this can also help with the absorption of calcium.
Folate (B9)	Dark green leafy vegetables, beans, peanuts, sunflower seeds, fresh fruits and whole grains.	Folic acid, also known as folate, is essential for forming DNA and plays a crucial role in breaking down protein and producing healthy red blood cells. Signs of low levels include anaemia, weight loss, weakness, headaches and it is a risk factor for heart disease. It can also help reduce hot flushes, which are a common symptom of menopause.
Omega-3	Oily fish – SMASH: sardines, mackerel, anchovies, salmon, herrings – tinned, fresh or frozen. Aim for 2–3 palm-size servings per week.	A long-chain fatty acid that your body can't produce, so we must include it in our diet. Crucial for every cell in your body, as well as being anti-inflammatory and key for brain health. If you don't eat fish, it may be worth looking into a good supplement. Make sure it contains the two most important types of omega-3 – EPA and DHA.
Magnesium	Almonds, green leafy vegetables, black beans, avocado, pumpkin seeds, whole grains and dark chocolate. In addition, add Epsom salts to your evening bath and soak for 20 minutes to help the salts absorb.	Magnesium is an important mineral. It can help improve mood and promote healthy bones and hormone levels. It is also important for energy production and sleep.

CHAPTER 15

Unpacking UPFs: What's Really on Your Plate?

There was a time when I thought I was making smart choices. I'd grab a healthy snack bar between sessions, throw together a quick wrap with supermarket hummus, and call it a win if the word protein or high fibre appeared on the label. But as I started looking more closely, especially after seeing how many of my clients felt bloated, foggy or fatigued despite eating what they *thought* was a balanced diet, I realised that something wasn't adding up.

Ultra-processed foods (UPFs) have become so normal that many of us don't even realise how often we're eating them. They're dressed up in language that makes us feel like we're doing something good for ourselves, but they're usually doing the opposite. If you've ever felt like you're doing everything right but still can't shift the brain fog, the bloating, the crashes and the cravings, UPFs could be the reason why.

UPFs are foods that have been significantly altered from their original form. They often contain additives, emulsifiers, flavour enhancers, artificial sweeteners, preservatives and other substances you'd never have in your kitchen. But they also hide behind slick packaging and healthy branding.

Things like:

- low-fat yoghurts with added thickeners and sweeteners
- protein or cereal bars with endless ingredients
- supermarket sauces with stabilisers and colourants
- bread with a shelf life of 2 weeks
- plant-based meat alternatives packed with artificial flavourings

While they can seem harmless or even healthy, they affect how we feel, function and age.

The science is catching up to what many of us have long felt in our bodies. Studies from Europe and beyond have shown that diets high in UPFS are linked to increased risks of cardiovascular disease, type 2 diabetes, cognitive decline, depression and early mortality.[51]

It's not just what these foods contain but what they lack. Fibre, essential nutrients and natural compounds that protect our cells are often stripped away or never present in the first place. The result? A body that's undernourished, inflamed and running on borrowed time.

UPFs can also interfere with the gut microbiome, that vast and delicate ecosystem that influences everything from mood and immunity to hormone balance and longevity. For women in midlife, when oestrogen levels begin to shift and inflammation creeps in more easily, this disruption can feel even more intense.

Why It Hits Harder in Midlife

Here's the thing: what you could once get away with, you can't anymore. You feel it. A couple of processed meals might leave you tired for days. A few too many artificial sweeteners and your sleep's off, your gut's in knots, your mood's unpredictable.

Our changing hormonal landscape means we're more sensitive to blood sugar spikes and dips. Our joints are more vulnerable to inflammation. Our brains are more reactive to the chemicals and additives we never used to think twice about. And because midlife is also when stress is often peaking – family pressures, work demands and ageing parents – it's easy to default to what's convenient.

But convenient shouldn't mean compromising your future health.

It's tempting to demonise UPFs, but this chapter isn't about shame. It's about awareness and gentle shifts. There's no judgement if you've relied on convenience: life is busy and food is emotional. But knowledge gives you back your power.

When you know what UPFs are and how they work, you can start to notice their presence and slowly, consistently, make other choices. It doesn't mean eliminating every packet in your cupboard overnight. It means becoming more discerning. Getting curious. Finding real pleasure in real food again.

Simple, Sustaining Alternatives

When women in my community begin to move away from UPFs, they often expect to feel deprived. But instead, they feel *relief*. Their digestion improves, their energy stabilises and their sleep deepens. And many describe something even more profound: a sense of coming back to themselves.

You don't need complicated swaps or trendy ingredients. A tin of wild salmon, a handful of baby spinach, a spoonful of olive oil and a few toasted seeds make a better wrap filling than anything in a healthy supermarket sandwich. Roasted chickpeas can become your new go-to snack. Real yoghurt, real fruit, a drizzle of honey – it's food your body understands. Food your body trusts.

Reducing UPFs isn't about restriction. It's about raising your standard for what goes into your body, because you understand the value of what it gives you back.

You don't need to fear food. You just need to feel empowered around it. And when you do, that power ripples out into your family, your friendships, your future. Because when you eat well, you live well. And when you live well, you age on your own terms.

CHAPTER 16

Rethinking Alcohol's Role in a Long Life

I recall the first time I watched *Live to 100: Secrets of the Blue Zones*. Their secrets seemed simple: plant-based diets, natural movement, close community and purpose. But one detail made me pause: in some areas, they drank alcohol daily.

Dan Buettner, the researcher behind the Blue Zones, noted that many of these long-living populations shared wine with meals, often among friends or family. In Sardinia, a glass of local Cannonau red wine, rich in antioxidants, was part of daily life. Buettner cited studies suggesting that moderate drinkers outlived both heavy drinkers and abstainers. And yet, despite all my admiration for his work, this is the one area that gives me pause.

While the image of a long table under the sun, surrounded by laughter and a glass of wine, is idyllic, it doesn't reflect how most people drink today.

Let's be clear, people in Blue Zones don't drink like many of us do in modern life. In Sardinia or Ikaria, wine is typically consumed in small quantities, paired with food and rarely on its own. It's not about wine o'clock at the end of a stressful day or binge-drinking on weekends. It's tied to tradition, connection and a slower pace of living.

This is important because it suggests that it may not be the alcohol itself that's beneficial but the way it's consumed: with people, in moderation, alongside whole foods, in a relaxed setting.

But what does the research say?

While early observational studies hinted that moderate alcohol intake might reduce the risk of heart disease or promote longevity,[52] more recent, large-scale studies found no evidence that moderate alcohol consumption conferred health benefits. The safest level of drinking appeared to be none at all.

Public health organisations are now taking a firmer stance. The World Health Organization and even the UK's Chief Medical Officer state that there's no completely safe level of alcohol use, especially when it comes to cancer risk.

So, how do we make sense of this?

It is possible that earlier studies were biased. Moderate drinkers often had higher incomes, better access to healthcare and stronger social connections, factors that independently boost longevity. Meanwhile, abstainers sometimes included those who had quit drinking due to illness, making the data misleading.

From a midlife health perspective, particularly for women navigating perimenopause or menopause, alcohol is even more complex. While a glass of wine might feel like a moment of calm, it's worth understanding what's happening under the surface:

- **Hormonal disruption:** Alcohol can affect oestrogen metabolism, often worsening symptoms like hot flushes, mood swings and sleep disturbances.
- **Sleep interference:** Alcohol may help you fall asleep initially, but it disrupts REM sleep, leading to poorer quality rest and early waking.

- **Increased anxiety:** Many women find themselves trapped in the anxiety loop, using alcohol to relax, but waking up feeling more on edge.

- **Weight gain and insulin resistance:** Alcohol is metabolised differently than food, often leading to increased abdominal fat and disrupted blood sugar balance.

- **Gut health:** Alcohol alters the microbiome, inflames the gut lining, and can worsen digestive issues.

And while the occasional glass may seem harmless, the cumulative impact can be significant, especially during a phase of life when our bodies are already undergoing changes.

We don't need alcohol to live longer or live better. The true longevity boosters from the Blue Zones are available to all of us, with or without the wine:

- **Moving naturally:** Walking, gardening, dancing, movement woven into daily life.

- **Plant-based eating:** Beans, grains, leafy greens and whole foods at the centre of the plate.

- **Community:** Spending time with people who lift you.

- **Purpose and joy:** Waking with a reason to get up in the morning.

I've thought a lot about where I stand on this. Alcohol is one area we can let go of without sacrificing any of the benefits of a long life. Letting it go might enhance your energy, clarity, sleep and self-trust in ways that truly ripple through your life. I will encourage you to do this when you follow the plan, giving yourself the best opportunity for success.

This isn't about being perfect. It's about being intentional. If alcohol has become a habitual part of your life, I gently invite you to examine why. Is it for connection? Relaxation? Reward? And could those needs be met in other, more nourishing ways?

Connection doesn't have to come in a glass. I gave up alcohol for 2 years and rarely drink now. Whether it's herbal tea, kombucha, sparkling water with lime or a homemade mocktail, I can still clink glasses, share stories and mark life's moments without compromising my health.

So, here's my invitation to you: reflect on your relationship with alcohol. Be curious, not critical. If it's serving you, great. If it's not, know that you're not alone and that the most powerful habit shifts often begin with a single, honest moment of awareness.

Weight-Loss Injections: Friends, Foes or Fixes?

I was sitting on the fence about this one, but the conversations are happening, and this is the right place to address it. Let me start by saying this: I completely understand the pull of a quick fix. When you've been battling your weight, your energy, your self-worth, and your body feels like it's working against you, it's no wonder that weight-loss medications like Ozempic or Wegovy feel like a lifeline. And for some, they genuinely are.

These GLP-1 medications, originally designed to treat type 2 diabetes, have shown impressive results in supporting weight loss and improving metabolic markers like blood sugar and cholesterol. As we know, excess visceral fat and insulin resistance are major drivers of chronic disease and reduced lifespan, so they may have a role to play in the longevity conversation.

But here's where I believe the conversation needs to evolve.

We're in the early days of truly understanding what weight-loss medications mean for long-term health. We don't yet know how sustained use will affect things like muscle preservation, bone density, mental well-being or even how people cope once they come off them. We know that when you build your health from the ground up through strength training, nutrient-dense food, sleep, stress management and genuine self-connection, you're laying the most powerful foundation there is.

And I've seen this in real time.

Take Rachel. She joined my Owning Your Menopause programme after using semaglutide (a form of weight-loss injections) for 6 months. She'd lost weight, yes, but she felt weaker, more anxious and unsure of how to move forward. The medication had helped reduce her appetite, but it hadn't taught her how to eat in a way that nourished her body, nor how to trust it. She'd lost muscle along with fat, and her energy was flat.

Over the next 12 weeks, we focused on rebuilding her relationship with movement and food. We started small, adding protein to her meals, strength training twice weekly, improving her sleep and carving out time for herself. She reconnected with what her body was capable of. We also discussed the why behind her goals: weight loss, strength, energy, independence and confidence.

Fast-forward 6 months and Rachel is no longer using the medication. Her weight is stable. But more importantly, she feels empowered. She trusts her habits. She's gaining lean muscle. Her blood markers look better than ever. And she told me recently, 'I didn't realise how much of myself I'd handed over to the drug. Now I feel like I'm back in the driver's seat.'

I share this not to diminish the potential value of these medications; they offer a critical stepping stone for many. But they are just that: a *step*, not the destination. The magic happens when we shift from outsourcing our health to truly owning it.

That's what I want for you. Whether or not medication is part of your journey, let's make sure you are at the centre of it.

PART 2.3
Mental Well-Being

When we discuss longevity, the conversation often starts with what we can see and measure: fitness levels, cholesterol readings, blood pressure and body composition. Concentrating on tangible aspects is easy: moving more, eating better and sleeping soundly. However, true longevity isn't merely about living longer; it's about the quality of those years. It's about how alive we feel while we live them. Central to that is mental health.

The mind is not separate from the body; it is its constant companion, quietly shaping how we move through the world. A strong, flexible mind helps us navigate stress and uncertainty while also empowering us to find joy, stay connected and maintain a sense of meaning, factors now proven to contribute as much to a long life as diet or exercise. Longevity research increasingly indicates that our thinking, connections and coping mechanisms profoundly impact how we age physically and emotionally.[53]

Stress, loneliness and a lack of emotional regulation don't just feel uncomfortable; they cause physiological changes. Prolonged mental strain elevates cortisol, shortens telomeres (the protective caps at the ends of our DNA) and increases systemic inflammation. Over time, these changes heighten our vulnerability to conditions such as cardiovascular disease, cognitive decline, type 2 diabetes and autoimmune disorders. Chronic psychological distress becomes a silent accelerator of ageing.

On the other hand, emotional resilience – a mental muscle we can all strengthen – acts as a buffer. By cultivating inner calm, nurturing perspective and remaining emotionally agile, we help reduce stress-related inflammation and support a more balanced hormonal environment.

Another equally powerful predictor of longevity is connection. In one of Harvard's longest-running studies on human happiness and health, researchers found that close relationships – more than money, fame or genetics – keep people healthy and fulfilled as they grow older.[54] It's not about the number of friends or the frequency of social events, but the quality of connection: feeling truly seen, valued and supported.

And if there's one thing midlife has taught me both personally and through the thousands of women I've worked with, it's this: we cannot keep pouring from an empty cup and expect to feel well.

So much of the health space focuses on doing more: eating this, moving like that, taking this supplement, tracking, measuring and optimising. And yes, all of those things can have a place. However, when we focus solely on action, we overlook the deeper truth. True vitality comes when we learn to slow down and tune back in.

This part of the book is also about what happens when we allow ourselves to rest.

Let me be clear: this didn't come naturally to me. I've always been a doer. A planner. Someone who pushes through. But that approach only got me so far. When my own body began to shift when hormones changed, when sleep became more elusive, when I found myself wired but exhausted, I had to rethink what thriving looked like.

That's when these tools became essential:

- Journalling gave me space to process the messiness of it all without judgement. It helped slow my racing thoughts, process emotions and created a sense of clarity and control.
- Music became a powerful way to shift my mood when motivation felt flat.
- Rest helped me reframe recovery not as laziness, but as a form of strength.

Navigating poor sleep in perimenopause and beyond has been a journey in itself, one that has taught me the importance of supporting our body's natural rhythms, rather than fighting against them.

And lastly, let's not forget joy. Often overlooked in conversations about health, joy is more than a fleeting emotion; it's a state of vitality. Experiencing joy, wonder and laughter activates healing pathways in the body. It nourishes the nervous system, enhances heart rate variability and restores balance. Making space for joy is not self-indulgent; it's life-sustaining.

CHAPTER 17

Hormones, Ageing and Mental Resilience

For years, I underestimated just how much my hormones influenced my mental resilience. I always believed that if I exercised regularly, ate well and kept a positive mindset, I could power through any emotional storm, stress, fatigue or overwhelm. And for a long time, that worked. But as I moved through different life stages, I began to realise that my emotional well-being wasn't always something I could will into balance. There were forces at play inside my body, hormonal shifts that carried far more weight than I'd given them credit for.

Like many women, I first got a glimpse of hormonal influence during my teenage years. Those rollercoaster moods before my period, the anxiety, the emotional sensitivity, they were all early signs of the fluctuating levels of oestrogen and progesterone. But back then, it was just brushed off as hormones, nothing to really explore or understand. It wasn't until I entered perimenopause that those familiar feelings returned, amplified and more persistent, catching me off guard.

Brain fog, random surges of anxiety and sleepless nights became a regular feature. At first, I thought I was just more stressed than usual. But it didn't feel like typical stress. It was as though my brain and emotions were operating on a frequency I couldn't quite control. That's when I started digging deeper and discovered how much hormonal change was shaping my internal world.

Oestrogen

Oestrogen, it turns out, had been one of my brain's greatest allies until it started to fade. I don't know about you, but I felt sharp, capable and emotionally steady when my oestrogen levels were consistent. As they began to dip, though, I started feeling like a stranger to myself. I was more irritable, quicker to snap and found myself stuck in spirals of self-doubt that I hadn't experienced before.

Reading about oestrogen's role in serotonin production was a lightbulb moment.

Serotonin

The neurotransmitter that helps us feel good, calm, and emotionally stable depends on oestrogen to work properly. So, when oestrogen drops (whether it's before your period or during the perimenopausal transition), so does serotonin. It made complete sense. This wasn't weakness or poor coping skills. This was a physiological shift and one that, once I understood, I could begin to work with instead of feeling defeated by.

Progesterone

If oestrogen was the energy and mood-supporting hormone, progesterone was the calm in the storm. I hadn't really noticed its presence until it began to disappear. Suddenly, my once peaceful sleep was broken up by 3 a.m. wake-ups, racing thoughts and a body that just couldn't unwind. The daytime impact was just as frustrating: heightened anxiety, irritability and a sense of emotional edge I couldn't shake.

Learning that progesterone enhances GABA, our brain's natural calming chemical, explained a lot. Without enough of it, the body's ability to wind down, relax and let go is compromised. I knew I couldn't stop these hormonal changes, but I also knew I could support myself through them. I began focusing more on my sleep hygiene, things like regular magnesium intake, a calming evening routine and mindfulness techniques to help settle my nervous system before bed. These weren't magic fixes, but they gave me a sense of agency again.

Cortisol

I'd always been proud of my ability to manage stress. I could juggle multiple roles, push through when I was tired and still show up for everyone else. But behind the scenes, cortisol, the stress hormone, was slowly wearing me down. I didn't even realise how much it had built up until I found myself constantly wired but exhausted, emotionally depleted and overwhelmed by even small things.

Women are more sensitive to stress hormones than men, and oestrogen helps buffer cortisol's effects. As oestrogen declines, so does our resilience to stress. What once felt manageable started to feel like too much. That's when I knew I had to shift how I approached stress. I brought in practices like meditation, journalling, deep breathing and something I hadn't done enough of: self-compassion. I also reassessed my relationship with exercise. While I loved high-intensity workouts, I began to see how too much of them could spike my cortisol even more. Strength training and daily walks became my foundation, helping me stay strong without tipping my stress levels over the edge.

Oxytocin

One of the biggest surprises in my hormonal journey was how deeply I craved connection during times of hormonal fluctuation. I've always enjoyed my own company, but suddenly, I found solitude harder to sit with. I wanted warmth, kindness, understanding – something more than just surface-level interactions.

That's when I learnt about oxytocin, the love and connection hormone. It's released during positive social interactions, hugs, acts of kindness and even meaningful conversation. And crucially, it helps counteract stress and anxiety. During challenging hormonal transitions, seeking out supportive relationships wasn't just a nice-to-have, it was essential. I made a conscious effort to spend time with people who lifted me up, and I prioritised quality connections over quantity. It changed everything.

Testosterone

While testosterone is often seen as a male hormone, it plays a vital role in women's lives, too, impacting energy, confidence and motivation. There's still a lot we don't fully understand about how testosterone fluctuations affect women during midlife, but what we do know is that strength training and maintaining an active lifestyle seem to help. For me, it was another reminder that moving my body purposefully wasn't just about the muscle, it was about mindset too.

The biggest lesson I've learnt through all of this is that mental resilience isn't about muscling through or pretending everything is fine. It's about learning to listen, adjust and meet yourself with kindness. Some days, that means pushing forward with focus and energy. Other days, it means resting without guilt, pausing without shame and understanding that slowing down is part of the process.

Working with my hormones instead of against them has been one of the most empowering shifts in my life. It's helped me navigate life's transitions with more grace, patience and a deeper sense of connection to myself. I no longer feel like I'm battling my body. I'm learning to support it with movement, nourishing food, rest and the company of people who remind me that I'm not alone.

If you're navigating a similar chapter, please hear this: you are not broken, you are not alone and you are not powerless. Hormones will shift, but you can continue to thrive with awareness and the right tools.

CHAPTER 18

How Exercise Positively Influences the Mind for Longevity

When people think of exercise, they often picture toned muscles, heart health or fitting into a certain size. But behind the physical changes lies something even more powerful: what movement does for the mind. In every life stage, and especially in midlife and beyond, regular movement is one of the most effective ways to build emotional strength, reduce anxiety and feel more grounded.

Mental resilience isn't just about pushing through; it's about learning how to bounce back, stay present and support the mind as much as the body. Movement plays a critical role in that. I notice a huge shift in mental clarity after exercise. Brain fog lifts, thoughts feel more organised and a sense of calm often follows, even after a short walk or a strength session. From doing research and my own understanding, this is more than just anecdotal; it's deeply biological.

Exercise boosts brain chemicals

Exercise increases the production of brain chemicals like serotonin, dopamine and endorphins, all of which play a role in mood regulation, motivation and stress response. These chemical shifts can act as natural antidepressants and anxiolytics, which is why movement is so often prescribed as part of mental health treatment plans.

In midlife, when hormonal fluctuations can leave many women feeling mentally foggy, emotionally overwhelmed or simply not themselves, this natural boost becomes even more valuable. The act of moving gently helps the brain find balance again.

Strength training for stability

Strength training in particular offers a unique mental benefit. Beyond building muscle, it creates a sense of stability and confidence, especially important in seasons of life when many things feel uncertain or in flux. For women navigating menopause or ageing-related changes, strength training supports not only bone and metabolic health but also emotional regulation. Lifting weights or performing resistance exercises has been shown to lower cortisol levels (the stress hormone), enhance sleep and improve focus. It also creates a sense of mastery – setting and achieving goals in a tangible, empowering way. It's not about lifting heavy or performing perfectly. It's about showing up consistently and gradually building physical and emotional strength in tandem.

Movement for stress

Hormonal shifts can also intensify the stress response. Declining oestrogen, for instance, reduces the brain's buffer against cortisol, making stress feel more intense and longer-lasting. Movement helps manage this. Rhythmic, repetitive activities like walking, swimming, cycling and strength circuits are especially effective. They activate the parasympathetic nervous system – our rest-and-digest state – helping bring the body out of stress and into recovery mode. This makes regular movement a kind of emotional reset button.

Rest might be best

On difficult days, it's not always about pushing through with intensity. Sometimes, it's the gentlest movements – like stretching, mobility work or a slow walk – that have the biggest impact. Consistency is what counts, not intensity.

Movement and friendship

One of the lesser talked-about mental benefits of movement is its ability to foster connection. Whether it's a shared class, a walking group or even an online workout community, moving with others promotes the release of oxytocin, the hormone associated with bonding, trust and emotional safety. In times when stress and hormonal changes can feel isolating, this connection is powerful. It reminds us we're not alone. That someone else gets it. That support is available often in the most unexpected places, like a friendly nod during a class or a shared laugh over a missed step. Social movement not only enhances mood but also reinforces resilience by strengthening a sense of belonging and joy.

Mental resilience isn't something anyone is born with; it's something we develop, one choice at a time. Regularly moving the body builds this resilience layer by layer. It's not about never struggling; it's about creating a toolkit that helps you navigate the struggle.

That's why movement remains one of the most accessible and powerful tools we have. Whether it's strength training to feel grounded and capable, walking to clear the mind, or stretching to release tension, exercise offers a meaningful way to reconnect with yourself. The 21-Day Plan is built around this principle. It's not about doing more, it's about doing what matters, with intention. Each day is thoughtfully designed to build strength, support your nervous system and restore balance physically and emotionally. By combining mobility, resistance and restorative practices, the plan helps you cultivate resilience, clarity and confidence. And as you begin to feel the shift – more focused, more steady, more like yourself – movement transforms from a task into a tool for living with strength and ease.

CHAPTER 19

Connection and Purpose for Longevity

Studies show that people with strong social ties tend to live longer, experience fewer chronic diseases, and enjoy greater emotional well-being.[55] Conversely, loneliness and social isolation are associated with an increased risk of heart disease, depression, cognitive decline and even early death.

Loneliness isn't just a feeling; it's a physical health risk. Research has found that chronic loneliness can be as harmful as smoking 15 cigarettes a day. Loneliness:

- raises cortisol (the stress hormone)
- increases inflammation
- weakens the immune system
- accelerates ageing

The impact is stark. Social isolation is associated with:

- high blood pressure
- obesity
- anxiety
- depression
- increased risk of dementia

However, even simple acts of kindness or shared laughter can mitigate these effects, fostering meaningful interactions. When we engage socially, our bodies release oxytocin, the hormone that promotes bonding, which in turn lowers stress, boosts immunity and supports cardiovascular health. And the benefits ripple out: people with good support systems are more likely to exercise, eat well and take care of their health.

I've seen the power of connection in my own life. My mother, now in her seventies, thrives because of the friendships and community she's nurtured. She joins clubs, organises events and maintains a strong sense of purpose. In contrast, an elderly neighbour who lives alone has slowly withdrawn from the world. Though physically capable, the lack of interaction has taken a visible toll on his mental and emotional well-being.

The difference is clear: social engagement keeps us vibrant, while isolation dims our spark.

Supportive relationships also provide a critical foundation for emotional resilience. Life brings inevitable challenges – loss, illness, transitions – but those with a strong support network are better equipped to cope, recover and grow. Sharing worries, being heard and receiving encouragement from trusted people can make the difference between sinking under stress or rising with strength. One friend, for example, lost her husband in her fifties. For a time, she retreated inward. But by leaning on her social circle and reconnecting with her community, she found strength, joy and a renewed sense of purpose.

Connection matters. In the Blue Zones, older adults don't fade into inactivity; they stay engaged, mentor younger generations, contribute to their communities and remain active in ways that suit their strengths. Research shows that a sense of purpose lowers stress, supports brain health and reduces the risk of chronic disease. In my work with midlife and older women, I've consistently seen that those who maintain hobbies, volunteer, mentor or create – even in small ways – radiate vitality. On the other hand, losing a role or identity after retirement or family transitions can leave people adrift. Reconnecting with a sense of purpose can reignite energy and meaning.

How to Reconnect

The beauty of social connection is that it's always within reach. Whether deepening existing relationships, forming new ones or finding a new purpose in daily life, intentional actions can profoundly benefit well-being.

- **Superficial small talk is common, but deeper conversations form lasting bonds.** Asking meaningful questions, listening without distraction and showing genuine interest create trust and intimacy. Vulnerability is also key; being open about your own experiences invites others to do the same, fostering mutual understanding and support.

- **People may not remember everything you say, but they always remember how you made them feel.** Being present, kind and curious can transform relationships powerfully.

- **Communities offer natural places to build these connections.** From fitness classes and book clubs to choirs, volunteering groups and faith communities, shared activities provide structure, purpose and social support. Consistency helps. The more often you show up, the easier it becomes to develop friendships that last. One newly retired client who felt isolated joined a local walking group. What started as a way to stay active soon became her social lifeline: an outlet for laughter, shared stories and connection. Another woman in her sixties joined a strength training class and formed lifelong friendships with other like-minded women. Together, they travel, support one another and uplift their community.

- **Some of the most enriching relationships come from outside our age group.** Older adults have wisdom and life experience to share, while younger people bring fresh energy and perspective. Intergenerational connections can offer a deep sense of meaning.

- **Mentorship, tutoring and community volunteering allow for mutual growth and can restore purpose after major life changes.** In my own family, after losing her partner, my mother rediscovered connection through bridge and music, which eventually led her to organise concerts and even find love again. Her story is a reminder that new chapters are always possible. Mentoring, teaching or simply spending time with younger relatives also helps build connections between generations, enhancing both emotional resilience and social identity.

- **One of the most powerful ways to cultivate meaning is by contributing to something larger than yourself.** Acts of kindness, both big and small, foster joy, reduce stress and enhance longevity. Volunteering for causes close to your heart, checking in on a neighbour or offering support to a friend can strengthen the fabric of your community and enhance your own sense of belonging. Sharing skills, providing mentorship or leading a group can reignite a sense of purpose that may have faded.

And just like with movement, connection and contribution are habits. The more you practise them, the more natural and fulfilling they become.

It's never too late to deepen a connection or rediscover a purpose. A long, vibrant life isn't only about adding years; it's about filling those years with joy, relationships, meaning and contribution. So, reach out. Be curious. Say yes to something new. Whether it's a conversation, a community project or rekindling an old friendship, every small step towards connection strengthens your mind and heart.

Your future self will thank you for it.

CHAPTER 20

Journalling

If you'd told me years ago that putting pen to paper could help me live a longer, healthier life, I might have raised an eyebrow. However, as I have explored the science of longevity and the power of sustainable habits, one thing has become crystal clear: journalling is a simple yet profoundly transformative tool. I also had no idea there were so many ways one could journal, which you will see later in this chapter.

For many women, the idea of journalling is appealing in theory but overwhelming in practice. It can feel too time-consuming, too emotional or like something reserved for poets, writers or people with more time. There's often a fear of doing it wrong or pressure to write something profound. But journalling isn't about being a good writer. It's not a school assignment. No one is marking your grammar. It's simply a check-in with yourself, a quiet space to pause and listen. Journalling provides that space. A way to take swirling thoughts out of your head and place them somewhere safe.

This practice offers more than stress relief. It builds awareness. Over time, journalling helps you:

- understand emotional patterns
- recognise triggers and energy shifts
- clarify what enhances your well-being
- tune into what you need
- develop self-compassion

It's like having a conversation with the wisest part of yourself, the part that often gets drowned out in the noise of daily life. No judgement or problem-solving, just letting it all out.

One of the most liberating things about journalling is that there is no set formula. You don't need 30 minutes or a beautiful notebook. Even a few words scribbled on the back of a receipt can be enough.

Throughout this book, we've discussed how small, consistent habits shape long-term health. Journalling fits within this framework. It strengthens emotional regulation, sharpens self-awareness and boosts mental resilience – essential qualities for a long and vibrant life.

I believe that journalling has helped me:

- process emotions in a constructive way
- reduce overwhelm and improve decision-making
- track physical symptoms and lifestyle habits
- reconnect with my values and purpose

When your mind feels overwhelmed, journalling helps clear the clutter. It's a way to mentally declutter and organise your thoughts. That clarity supports better decision-making and reduces cognitive overload, especially during hormonally intense times.

It's also a judgement-free space for emotional release. Women are often conditioned to keep emotions contained. But unexpressed anger, sadness or anxiety can damage health over time. Journalling provides a healthy outlet for releasing and reframing those feelings, thereby building emotional resilience. As someone diagnosed with ADHD later in life, it has also helped me understand myself more deeply. It's made me more forgiving, more curious and more capable of noticing patterns I used to miss.

Putting things on paper has been invaluable for tracking health-related habits. I've used it to track movement, nutrition and sleep, gaining valuable insights into what works best for my body. This tracking becomes especially empowering in midlife when our needs are changing.

Taking a moment before bed has also been a game-changer for sleep. By reflecting on what I'm thankful for, I calm my mind and fall asleep more easily. Since sleep is such a cornerstone of longevity, this slight shift has had a significant effect on my well-being.

Writing activates and preserves brain function – crucial as we age. Women, in particular, face a higher risk of cognitive decline due to hormonal changes. Journalling helps keep the brain engaged and thinking clearly, even during stressful seasons, and has also powerfully shifted my perspective. After losing my dad, I found it hard to feel grateful; even now, I struggle at times. But writing down what I am thankful for helps me focus on what I do have in the present.

One of journalling's greatest strengths lies in its adaptability. Whether you want to process emotions, stay accountable to your goals or simply make sense of a noisy mind, journalling can meet you exactly where you are.

Below are some of the most popular types of journalling, each offering something unique to support your long-term health journey. We will be focusing on Health and Habit Journalling when it comes to the Plan, but I feel it is good to have an understanding of all the ways one could journal in the future. Once you've established the habit, you can start experimenting and find the one that suits you best.

Reflective Journalling

Reflective journalling is one of the most grounding ways to reconnect with yourself. It offers a quiet space to pause and reflect on your day or week. Not to replay everything in detail, but to notice what stood out. Maybe it was a moment that lifted your spirits, something that made you feel uneasy or a conversation that stayed with you longer than expected. This kind of journalling helps you make sense of what's going on beneath the surface. It gives your thoughts and emotions a place to land, rather than letting them swirl around in your head. It's about noticing how you responded to what life threw at you and gently exploring why.

Why it matters for longevity

When you develop the habit of regular reflection, you begin to understand yourself more clearly. You spot the patterns that support your well-being and those that quietly erode it. That kind of self-awareness enables you to make more informed decisions about your health, relationships and future. It also fosters emotional resilience, a quality we need more than ever in midlife, when change is often happening on multiple levels simultaneously. Reflective journalling strengthens that vital connection between mind and body, which is at the heart of lasting well-being.

Gratitude Journalling

Gratitude journalling is one of the simplest yet most powerful ways to change how you feel. It's about intentionally noticing what's going well, what's bringing you joy and what you might usually overlook in the rush of the day. It could be as small as the comfort of your morning coffee, a kind message from a friend or the feeling of fresh air on your face during a walk. Writing down just three things you're grateful for can start to rewire your brain to focus on what's working rather than what's missing. And on the days that feel heavy or chaotic, that slight shift in focus can make a big difference. Gratitude isn't about pretending everything is fine. There was a time, after losing my dad, when I couldn't feel grateful. Not really. Everything felt heavy, and even though I had a full life, I just couldn't see it. It was gratitude journalling done gently, with no pressure, that helped me shift. Writing down even one or two things I was thankful for began to open a crack in the heaviness. A moment of laughter. A text from one of my children. Tiny things that reminded me I was still living. Still here. Still supported. It reminded me that my dad would not want me to be like this.

Why it matters for longevity

Regular gratitude journalling has been shown to improve mood, support better sleep, reduce stress and increase overall life satisfaction. All of these benefits help regulate the nervous system, lower inflammation and create a more balanced internal environment for your body and mind to thrive. As we age, staying connected to moments of joy and appreciation becomes a powerful tool for maintaining emotional well-being and promoting long-term health.

Bullet Journalling

Bullet journalling is a beautifully flexible way to bring more clarity and structure into your life. It combines elements of planning, tracking and reflection in one place. Some people use it to stay on top of daily tasks, while others track habits such as hydration, movement, mood or sleep. You can make it as simple or as creative as you like.

The beauty of bullet journalling is that it helps make the invisible visible. When life feels scattered or overwhelming, seeing your thoughts, goals and progress laid out on the page can create a sense of order. It becomes your personalised well-being dashboard, helping you stay on track without the pressure of perfection.

Why it matters for longevity

Structure supports consistency, and consistency is what leads to long-term change. Bullet journalling helps you stay engaged with your health goals in a way that feels encouraging rather than rigid. It gives you daily touchpoints that reinforce your intentions, whether that's getting more sleep, managing stress or drinking more water. Over time, those small check-ins add up to significant shifts in how you feel and function.

Stream of Consciousness Journalling

Stream-of-consciousness journalling is where you let it all out. No structure, no plan, no editing. You simply write whatever comes to mind. It might start with 'I don't know what to write,' and lead you somewhere completely unexpected. The goal isn't to sound clever or make sense. It's to clear the clutter and allow your thoughts to move freely.

This type of journalling is beneficial when your mind feels full or restless. It provides a safe space to release unspoken thoughts, quiet worries or simply process what's happening beneath the surface. You don't need to hold back or tidy things up. You're simply giving yourself permission to feel and express without judgement. I had done this without realising it was a type of journalling until I researched this book, and this one feels easier for me. I don't overthink it.

Why it matters for longevity

Holding on to stress and emotion can weigh heavily on the body. Over time, that internal tension can impact everything from sleep to digestion to immune function. Stream of consciousness journalling helps offload what you're carrying before it builds up. It supports emotional regulation, encourages self-compassion and can bring surprising clarity to situations you're stuck in. A few minutes of uncensored writing can leave you feeling lighter, calmer and more in control.

Morning Pages

Morning pages are a daily ritual where you write three full pages as soon as you wake up. The idea is to clear your head before the demands of the day set in. It doesn't matter what you write or how it sounds. This isn't for anyone else to read. It's simply a space to be honest, unfiltered and free. Some mornings it might feel like a brain dump. Other days, it might surprise you with insight or creativity. Either way, it gives you a sense of lightness and focus that can completely alter how you present yourself for the rest of the day. It's like clearing the mental cobwebs before you get dressed and get going.

Why it matters for longevity

How we start the day can shape everything that follows. Morning pages help reduce mental noise, lower stress levels and create space for calm and clarity. They're especially powerful during midlife when hormones, responsibilities and emotions often feel more intense. Taking just 10 to 15 minutes to write each morning can improve focus, support emotional wellbeing and help you respond to life with more intention rather than reactivity. Over time, this gentle habit can make a significant difference in how you feel, both mentally and physically.

Prompt-Based Journalling

Prompt-based journalling is ideal for those moments when you want to reflect but don't know where to start. It provides a simple question or statement to explore, such as 'What do I need more of right now?' or 'What am I ready to let go of?' These prompts gently guide your thinking and help you go deeper, especially when life feels busy or your thoughts feel muddled. You can use the same prompt regularly to track your growth or try new ones each week to spark reflection in different areas. The beauty of prompts is that they meet you exactly where you are, offering direction without pressure.

Why it matters for longevity

Taking time to explore meaningful questions helps you stay connected to your values, needs and direction. This connection can influence the choices you make around rest, movement, relationships and boundaries. In midlife, when so much is shifting, prompts can help you stay grounded in what matters most.

They also support emotional resilience and self-leadership, which are key for long-term well-being and creating a life that feels fulfilling, not just functional.

Health and Habit Journalling

Health and habit journalling is a practical tool that helps you keep track of what supports your body and mind each day. You might log your meals, energy levels, sleep patterns, movement, mood or symptoms. Over time, this builds a clear picture of how your lifestyle is affecting your overall well-being. This is what we will focus on over the 21 days, to keep it relatable and achievable.

Rather than aiming for perfection, this kind of journalling is about awareness. It helps you identify what's working, what's missing and where small changes can have a significant impact. You're not tracking to be rigid. You're tracking to understand and support yourself better.

Why it matters for longevity

When it comes to long-term health, small habits make a significant difference. This kind of journalling helps you stay connected to those habits and notice the patterns that might otherwise go unnoticed. It's especially useful as we age, when things like sleep, balance, strength, digestion and energy can change dramatically. By tracking your daily routines and responses, you become better equipped to make decisions that support long-term strength, balance and vitality.

Affirmation Journalling

Affirmation journalling is the practice of writing down positive, supportive statements that reflect who you are becoming or how you want to feel. These include being capable of adapting to change and having a strong body that gets stronger every day. It's about choosing your focus and shifting your inner dialogue to something more encouraging.

Writing affirmations helps reinforce self-belief, especially on days when doubt or comparison creeps in. You can repeat the same affirmation daily or create new ones based on what you need most that week. Over time, these statements begin to feel less like wishful thinking and more like grounded truth. Affirmations with kids are a great way to encourage resilience and self-belief.

Why it matters for longevity

The way we speak to ourselves shapes how we feel, how we act and even how our bodies respond to stress. Affirmation journalling helps interrupt the negative self-talk that can become so ingrained, particularly during midlife when confidence can take a hit. By regularly reinforcing positive messages, you strengthen your mindset and support a more balanced nervous system. Internal stability plays a decisive role in maintaining long-term physical and emotional health.

Visual Journalling

Visual journalling brings creativity into your well-being practice. Instead of relying only on words, you might use sketches, colour, shapes, collage or diagrams to express how you feel. It's not about being artistic. It's about allowing yourself to communicate differently, especially when thoughts or emotions feel too big, messy or unclear to put into sentences.

Some people combine drawings with notes or affirmations. Others use it as a calming, meditative practice without any writing at all. There's no right or wrong way to do it. The process itself is what's healing.

Why it matters for longevity

Creative expression supports emotional regulation and reduces stress, which has a direct impact on long-term health. It can also help unlock insights that get missed when we only process things logically. For those who feel overstimulated, stuck in their heads or disconnected from joy, visual journalling offers a gentle way back to self. It reminds us that healing, growth and expression can be colourful, intuitive and deeply personal.

Journalling is one of the simplest and most powerful ways to check in with yourself. It helps you slow down and honestly notice what's going on in your body, mind and day-to-day life. Whether you're jotting down things you're grateful for, tracking your sleep, working on mobility, balance, strength or letting out the jumble of thoughts in your head, journalling gives you space to breathe and reset.

And you don't have to do it perfectly. You don't even have to do it every day. What matters is that it becomes a space that feels like yours, a quiet corner of your routine where you can reflect, release pressure and reconnect with what's important to you. More importantly, you can feel the changes.

As we move into the 21-Day Plan, I want to reassure you that you do not need to write pages. That would be impossible, but I am inviting you to be more present. What I encourage is a short, flexible rhythm. In the morning, check in with how you feel, what you need and which habit you want to commit to. In the evening, note what you noticed, what helped and how you might support yourself better tomorrow.

We'll be using Health and Habit Journalling as a key part of building lasting change. This is where you'll start to notice what's really working for you: how your balance and strength are improving, whether it's more sleep, more movement, more water or simply more moments to breathe. It's not about being strict. It's about building awareness so you can make choices that feel good and support the life you want to live long term.

If you're new to journalling, start wherever you are. Be curious, not critical. Don't worry about how it looks or sounds. This isn't about doing more. It's about noticing more. Feeling more. Living more fully.

CHAPTER 21

Music for Motivation and Longevity

There's a reason the right song at the right time can change everything. Music can shift your energy, lift your mood and bring you straight back to yourself. It's not just entertainment, it's medicine for the mind and body. And when it comes to supporting motivation, resilience and longevity, it's a tool you can use daily.

Music can be used intentionally, especially in midlife, to help you move more easily, feel more emotionally balanced and start your day with purpose. The best part? You don't need any special skills or extra time. Just a song. A beat. A rhythm to remind you that you're alive, capable and ready to take up space.

Midlife is a season of transition. Hormonal shifts, emotional changes and lifestyle demands can make it harder to find motivation, especially first thing in the morning. Some days, even movement can feel like a mountain to climb.

Music helps. It lights up reward centres in the brain, stimulates dopamine (your motivation and get-up-and-go chemical) and reduces cortisol (the stress hormone that leaves you feeling heavy and foggy). The right music can move you physically and emotionally, whether walking, stretching, lifting or just trying to start the day with energy.

It's not about hype or intensity; it's about connection – the kind that makes you nod your head, tap your foot and remember who you are.

As part of the 21-Day Plan, you'll be encouraged to use music in your morning motivation ritual. Think of it as your energetic switch-on – a moment of rhythm and reset to start your day with intention.

I am going to be asking you to:

- Play a track or playlist that lifts your mood (you can use one of the suggested ones or create your own).

- Let the music move you – stretch, walk, breathe or even dance for a few minutes.

- Use the energy to begin your day feeling lighter, more present and more motivated.

This doesn't have to be formal or time-consuming. Just one or two songs can shift your entire mindset. The point is to let music become a signal.

Music isn't just background noise. It actively supports your body and brain in ways that matter for long-term health.

Listening to music can:

- Boost dopamine, supporting motivation, mood and memory.

- Lower cortisol, helping reduce stress and inflammation.

- Increase oxytocin, enhancing feelings of connection and safety.

- Improve focus and mental clarity when used during work or exercise.
- Trigger emotional release, helping process feelings that may be hard to express in words.
- Support brain plasticity, especially when paired with movement, helping maintain cognitive health over time.

If movement feels like a chore, pairing it with music can change your relationship with it. Music makes movement more enjoyable, more consistent and often more effective. It turns everyday activity into something that feels like self-expression, not just self-discipline.

Movement doesn't have to look a certain way to be effective. If it gets your body and your mood moving, it counts.

Your playlist should feel like you. It should include songs that energise, comfort, inspire or ground you. These tracks make you want to move, sing or simply smile.

You might want different playlists for different needs:

- Morning Energy Boost
- Strength & Power
- Walk & Reflect
- Wind Down & Stretch
- Mood Reset

I want you to start with one power song every morning or at times when you feel low that lifts you up.

Music connects us to who we were, who we are and who we're becoming. It helps us process emotions, connect with memories and feel part of something bigger. For many women in midlife, it becomes a portal to joy, nostalgia, empowerment or simply *presence*. Whether you sing, dance or quietly listen, music becomes a companion through change – one that doesn't judge, one that reminds you of your strength, your softness and your spirit.

And music is a free, accessible, beautiful tool that's always available. Use it as often as you like. Let it lift you when energy is low, soothe you when you're tense, and remind you daily that your body and mind are still deeply connected, capable and worthy of care.

So, press play. Move a little. Smile a little. Start your day with sound, rhythm and intention. Let music become your ally in this next chapter of longevity. You don't need to wait for motivation to arrive. You can create it. One song at a time.

CHAPTER 22

Rest and Recovery: Slowing Down to Thrive

Rest can feel like rebellion in a world that prizes busyness, pushing harder, doing more and constantly striving for progress. But to live long, vibrant lives, we must learn that longevity isn't just built in motion; it's built in pause. In the gentle exhale. In the quiet moments when the body isn't being pushed but instead being nurtured.

Many of us enter midlife having spent decades in a state of constant motion. We've raised families, built careers, cared for others and tried to stay fit and well along the way. We're conditioned to believe that doing equates to worth. So, it's no wonder that rest can feel foreign, maybe even uncomfortable. From personal experience, this is something, along with journalling, that I am trying hard to honour. I have seen many friends realise that rest isn't something to start once you're on the brink of burnout. It's a foundational part of the health and longevity journey. Without it, everything else you're doing, whether it's exercise, eating well or showing up for your people, will eventually start to fray at the edges.

Rest is where healing happens. It's the space in which your body repairs, your muscles grow, your hormones recalibrate and your mind processes. Without adequate recovery, your efforts can become counterproductive, leaving you exhausted, inflamed and wondering why things aren't clicking. When we honour rest, we step into a rhythm that supports long-term strength, resilience and clarity.

But the rest is more nuanced than simply getting more sleep. It has many faces, some subtle, some active, all essential.

There's physical rest, of course, the most obvious form. This includes the still, passive rest we get from sleep, stretching on the floor, lying down with your legs up the wall and letting your body soften into the moment. But physical rest can also be active: gentle walks, mobility work, breath-led yoga that keeps blood circulating and supports repair. For women in midlife, physical rest isn't about being idle, it's about offering the body a different kind of support. When hormones fluctuate and recovery slows, this kind of rest becomes even more vital. It's not a weakness to modify a workout or swap a high-intensity session for a walk in the woods. It's wisdom.

Then there is mental rest, which is often the first thing we lose in our hyperconnected world. Our brains are constantly fed by emails, notifications, decision-making, scrolling and multitasking. It's no wonder we often lie awake at night, our thoughts tangled in to-do lists and worries. Mental rest doesn't mean doing nothing, it means creating small, intentional pauses. A quiet moment with a cup of tea. Turning off your phone and letting your thoughts wander without interruption. These are not frivolous; they are restorative acts that allow the mind to soften, to untangle.

Emotional rest is something so many midlife women crave without even realising it. We've spent years being strong for others: holding space, offering support and masking our own overwhelm to keep the peace. But emotional rest is about releasing that mask.

It's being in the presence of someone you don't have to perform for. It's allowing yourself to cry, to be messy, to not have the answers. It's the exhale that comes when you admit, *I'm not okay right now,* and feel safe doing so. When we suppress emotion, we create inner tension that can manifest physically. Emotional rest invites release, and in that release, there is healing.

Sensory rest may sound unfamiliar, but once you notice sensory overload, you can't unsee it. The relentless brightness of screens, the background hum of traffic or TV, the constant buzz of alerts, it's all stimulation. Our nervous systems are rarely off-duty. Sensory rest means turning down the volume on the world. Dimming the lights in the evening. Lighting a candle instead of switching on overhead bulbs. Choosing silence over background noise. These are small shifts that have a profound effect on calming your system.

Then there's social rest – not isolation, but discernment. It's choosing who you spend time with based on how they make you feel. We all know the difference between being with someone who energises us and someone who depletes us. Social rest is stepping back from the performative, from the relationships that take more than they give. It's creating boundaries without guilt. It's allowing space for solitude so that when you do connect, it's meaningful.

What I've seen time and again is that when women begin to weave these layers of rest into their lives – not as emergency measures but as part of their daily rhythm – everything begins to shift. They move with more ease. Sleep improves. Cravings reduce. Strength returns. It's not always dramatic. Sometimes it's a subtle feeling: being a bit more patient, having a clearer mind, feeling more like yourself again.

Sally, a client in her late fifties, came to me feeling utterly stuck. She was eating well and exercising five times a week, but she felt constantly tired, sore and mentally foggy. She was frustrated that the energy she expected to gain from her efforts wasn't showing up. When we unpacked her routine, what we discovered was simple but powerful: she wasn't recovering. There was no space to breathe. No soft days. We pulled back on the intensity, built in rest days, added a bedtime routine and a 15-minute morning mobility flow. Within a month, her energy returned. Her body began responding again. She smiled more. She moved more freely. The missing link wasn't more effort, it was more ease.

You don't need to overhaul your life to start honouring rest. It begins with awareness: tuning in to when you're pushing past your limit, noticing the cues of fatigue before they become a shout. You can build rest into your day in small, sacred ways:

- A 10-minute walk without your phone.
- Five deep belly breaths before a meal.
- Turning off overhead lights and lighting a candle in the evening.
- Saying no without apology.
- Taking a nap without feeling guilty.
- Journalling what you feel, not just what you do.

In this 21-Day Plan, don't just focus on what you're doing, pay attention to how you're recovering. Progress isn't only measured in steps or strength gains. It's also in how well you sleep, how you manage stress and how often you feel at home in your own body.

Rest isn't passive. It's powerful. It's where your strength rebuilds, your clarity returns and your spirit reawakens. If movement is your momentum, recovery is your anchor. Together, they create the rhythm of a long, fulfilling life.

CHAPTER 23

Redefining Sleep for Longevity

Let's get one thing clear right from the start: sleep is important. But feeling guilty about not getting enough of it? That's often what does more damage than the missed hours themselves.

Midlife is rarely quiet. You're up late replying to emails, thinking about your children, ageing parents, your work or what on earth you're going to cook tomorrow. Perhaps you fall asleep exhausted, only to wake up at 3 a.m. with your mind racing and your body restless, and then spend the rest of the night in that frustrating twilight zone, neither asleep nor awake. And then comes the kicker: the internal dialogue. *Why can't I just sleep like I used to? What's wrong with me? How am I supposed to function today?*

This chapter is here to gently challenge that narrative. Yes, sleep is vital to our long-term health. However, striving for perfect sleep, or anything ideal, in a life that is anything but perfect, can be exhausting in itself. However, even small shifts can support your body's need for rest and build a foundation that will serve you for years to come.

As we age, sleep becomes more than a nightly recharge. It's when our brain clears out waste, when cells repair, hormones rebalance and our immune system gets a chance to recover. Sleep is your body's natural detox, reset and repair system. It's deeply protective against heart disease, diabetes, inflammation and cognitive decline. It plays a key role in reducing the risk of age-related diseases. But it doesn't have to be perfect to be effective. So, let's take the pressure off.

We've been sold the idea that unless you get 8 unbroken hours, it doesn't count. I don't think I have ever had that. Anyway, the good news is that that is not true. What matters most is the quality of your rest and how you support your body's natural rhythm throughout your day. It's also important to zoom out and see how sleep is connected to everything else you're already working on. Sleep doesn't stand alone. It's completely intertwined with the other pillars of longevity we're exploring in this book.

Take movement, for example. Gentle walking, strength training and daily activity all help regulate your circadian rhythm and release tension from the body, making it easier to fall into a more restorative sleep. On the other hand, poor sleep makes it harder to feel motivated to move, creating a cycle that's easy to get stuck in but also entirely possible to shift.

Nutrition also plays a crucial role. Blood sugar crashes caused by ultra-processed foods or late-night eating can disrupt your rest. Caffeine stays in the body much longer than most people realise, and even an afternoon coffee can hinder falling asleep. Foods high in magnesium, tryptophan and complex carbohydrates, such as oats, leafy greens, nuts and bananas, can gently encourage your nervous system into sleep mode. There's a synergy here that's worth noticing.

And then there's your gut. That fascinating, bacteria-rich ecosystem inside you has a direct connection to your brain. A thriving, well-fed microbiome helps regulate neurotransmitters like serotonin, which is the precursor to melatonin, the hormone that promotes sleep. So, if you've been working on gut health by adding fermented foods, more plants and more fibre, you're not just supporting digestion, you're also helping your sleep.

We also need to talk about mental well-being. How could we not? You already know how hard it is to sleep when your mind is in overdrive. Stress, anxiety and unprocessed thoughts all show up at night. But so do the tools to calm them. I have added journalling to the plan because practices like journalling before bed, listening to calming music or writing down your worries can all help quiet the noise and signal safety to your nervous system. Sometimes it's not that we can't sleep, it's that we haven't given ourselves permission to wind down.

A glass of wine in the evening can feel like a well-earned treat or even a coping mechanism for the overwhelm, but while it might help you fall asleep faster, as mentioned previously, alcohol is one of the biggest disruptors of deep, restorative rest. It fragments your sleep cycle, especially the REM stage, and increases night-time wake-ups. It also raises your heart rate, affects your breathing and can worsen hot flushes. I'm not here to tell you to never drink again, but it's worth being curious. If you're regularly waking up feeling unrefreshed or if your anxiety spikes the next day, try a few alcohol-free nights and see how your body responds. You might be surprised at the difference.

None of this is about perfection. You're not being marked on how well you sleep. You're tuning into your body and creating a space where rest is possible. That might involve adjusting your bedtime routine, keeping your bedroom cool or simply swapping late-night scrolling for 5 minutes of breathwork. And on those nights when nothing works and you still don't sleep well? That doesn't undo your progress. It just means tomorrow is another opportunity to try again.

Sleep is part of your long game. It supports your brain, heart, hormones, muscles and mood. It helps you process emotions and store memories. It keeps you steady, focused and resilient. It's one of the most protective tools you have, not just for the body you live in now, but for the body you want to carry you forward into later life. And part of owning your longevity is knowing that sometimes the best thing you can do isn't to force yourself to sleep but to trust that your body is doing its best, and to meet it with grace.

So tonight, instead of thinking I have to get 8 hours or else, what if you simply said, *I'm going to create the best conditions I can for rest, and whatever happens, I'll be okay.*

That's the energy we're bringing to sleep now. Gentle. Kind. Consistent. And completely in service of your future self.

PART 3

Assessing Your Health

Let's be honest, most of us don't wake up in the morning thinking, 'How's my balance today?' or wonder how strong our legs are compared to last year. But here's the thing: our ability to stand on one leg, get up from a chair, or even walk briskly without running out of breath tells us a lot about how well we'll move, function and thrive in the years ahead.

We often focus on weight, diet and exercise when we think about health. But there's something even more powerful that predicts long-term wellness: our functional fitness. The ability to balance, move easily and maintain strength in key muscle groups is directly linked to longevity, independence and overall well-being.

We take for granted the ability to move freely, confidently and without pain until we suddenly can't. Everyday actions, such as getting out of a chair, lifting a bag of groceries or climbing stairs, happen without thought until they don't. As discussed earlier, midlife changes bring shifts in strength, balance and mobility. The good news is that we have the power to influence how well we move and function as we age.

CHAPTER 24

The Importance of Functional Fitness

Functional fitness isn't about aesthetics or performance; it's about training to support real life. Unlike traditional gym workouts that isolate individual muscles, functional movements mimic the natural movements we make throughout the day. A squat isn't just an exercise; it's the ability to get up from the floor or a chair with ease. Lifting a weight overhead is similar to placing something on a high shelf. Carrying dumbbells is comparable to holding shopping bags or lifting a grandchild. These movements build the strength and stability needed to navigate daily demands confidently.

As previously mentioned, hormonal shifts during menopause accelerate muscle loss and weaken bones, increasing the risk of osteoporosis, joint pain and loss of strength. Without intervention, metabolism slows, coordination and balance decline, and movements that once felt effortless become harder. Functional fitness helps counteract these changes by preserving muscle mass, maintaining bone density and improving joint health.

Falling is one of the most significant risks associated with ageing. A simple loss of balance can result in fractures that drastically affect mobility and independence. Functional fitness improves stability through movements that challenge balance, strengthen the core and enhance reaction time. By regularly engaging in exercises that require shifting weight, standing on one leg or moving in multiple directions, we train our bodies to respond quickly and reduce the risk of falls.

Functional fitness also improves circulation, enhances brain function and reduces stress by releasing endorphins, which act as natural mood boosters. It plays a key role in reducing aches, pains and stiffness by keeping the body mobile and resilient. Posture improves, reducing strain on the lower back, shoulders and hips. And, perhaps most importantly, it fosters confidence in our ability to move, lift and carry on with life without limitations.

The beauty of functional fitness is its simplicity. It doesn't require a gym or complicated equipment. Getting up and down from the floor without using your hands is a powerful indicator of mobility and longevity. Carrying heavy objects helps build grip strength, which is linked to increased life expectancy. Squats, lunges and press-ups strengthen the body in ways that translate directly to everyday life. The goal isn't to master complex workouts but to move with intention, ensuring we can keep doing the things we love for years.

As we've explored throughout this book, longevity isn't just about lifespan, it's about healthspan. The choices we make today determine how well we age. Functional fitness is one of the most effective ways to future-proof our bodies, preserving independence and quality of life. It's not about chasing youth; it's about embracing strength at every stage, knowing that the work we put in now is an investment in the years ahead.

Seven movements for functional fitness

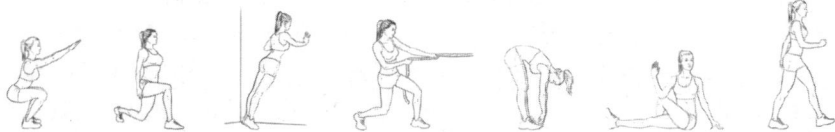

- **Squat**

The squat is one of the most complex movements the body can perform. It's important in daily life because a simple squat is comparable to sitting down and standing up. The muscles targeted are the glutes, core and quads.

- **Lunge**

Lunges are essential to lower body strength and stability. Many women feel off balance when they perform this move as their body is at a disadvantaged stance, as you put one foot in front of the other. This move demands excellent stability and balance. The lunge is a vital movement pattern that transfers well into walking, stair climbing and picking things up from the floor. Lunges will challenge your glutes, quads, core and hamstrings, and they use all three of those muscle groups more than a squat because of the split stance.

- **Push**

The push motion involves pushing something away from your body. This movement requires core and lower body stability. You may wonder why we need to focus on that movement pattern. Without realising it, you push yourself out of chairs and open doors, both of which require strength in your chest, triceps and shoulders.

- **Pull**

The pulling motion involves pulling something towards your body. For example, you may pull shopping bags over your shoulders, pull a car door shut or reach for things up high from the cupboard. This requires strength in your shoulders, chest, back and core.

- **Bend/Hinge**

We bend over to pick up things daily. Many women I see complain of lower back pain, which is often due to a weak posterior chain. The posterior chain consists of your hamstrings, glutes and lower back. So, we must focus on exercises that will help us strengthen this area. Making sure that we bend down properly and have the strength to do so are important when it comes to the hinge movement, which is one of the most functional daily movements.

- **Twist/Rotation**

All too often, we move more frequently in one plane. What I mean is we usually get up or down, moving forwards or backwards and from side to side. We do not often focus on twisting or rotation, which can cause many problems. Your core and obliques play a huge role in creating balance and stability. Being able to move in every direction can help prevent injuries.

- **Gait**

The ability to walk is a fundamental part of daily life and should be a priority and focus in any training programme. While this may seem obvious, it can form an excellent basis for beginners. Your gait is a combination of multiple movements.

CHAPTER 25

So, Where Are You Right Now?

In the following assessment, we will focus on cardiovascular endurance, muscle strength, flexibility and overall mobility.

To be able to measure your incremental improvements as we go through the 21-Day Plan, please complete these simple, science-backed tests before you start. The tests might seem basic, but trust me, they offer incredible insights into your body's resilience and where you might need to focus your efforts. They will form an integral part of the plan.

These predictive home longevity tests are highly beneficial because they give us insight into your functional fitness, mobility, balance and muscle strength – all crucial for maintaining independence, preventing falls and enhancing quality of life as we age. Studies consistently show that better performance on these tests correlates with lower mortality risk, reduced risk of injury and higher quality of life in later years. In the long term, regularly incorporating these exercise tests into a fitness routine will help maintain functional mobility and physical health, which are essential for longevity.

Mobility and Balance Tests:
Let's Assess Your Current Physical Health

To give you a clear picture of where you're starting from and how you're progressing, I've included seven simple longevity tests. These measure key areas linked to long-term health: strength, balance, mobility, flexibility, coordination and cardiovascular fitness.

You can complete all seven tests in one session (this is ideal) or spread them over a day or two if necessary. You'll need a stopwatch or timer (your phone is fine), a sturdy chair, a flat wall and a small, clear space.

Make a note of your results and retest every 7 days during the 21-Day Plan to track improvements and stay motivated.

1. Single Leg Stand Test

Why are we testing this? This simple yet powerful test assesses your balance and proprioception– your body's ability to sense its position in space without needing to look. These two elements are crucial for maintaining balance, coordination and confidence in movement.

As we age, proprioception naturally declines, leading to poorer balance.[56] This contributes to an increased risk of falls, reduced independence and even higher rates of mortality. Poor balance is a stronger predictor of longevity than many people realise.

Regularly practising this test doesn't just track your progress; it improves your balance, core strength, ankle stability and body awareness.

How to do it:
1. Stand barefoot near a wall or sturdy surface for safety.
2. Shift your weight onto one leg.
3. Lift the opposite foot off the floor, bending the knee to a 90-degree angle so that the thigh is parallel to the floor.
4. Start a timer as soon as your foot leaves the ground.
5. Hold for as long as you can without wobbling, touching the raised foot to the ground or using your hands or the wall for support.
6. Stop the timer when the balance is lost.
7. Repeat on the other leg.

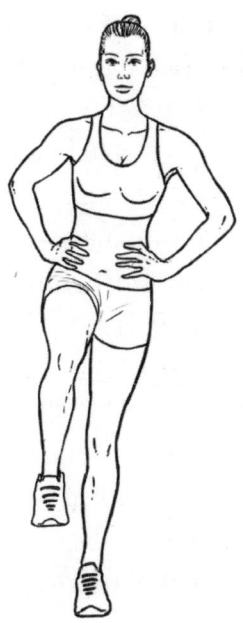

Progression tip: As your balance improves, try closing your eyes. This removes visual input, making the test far more challenging and engaging your deep stabilising muscles and proprioceptive awareness.

Goals and benchmarks: Use these general age-related benchmarks to see where you're starting from and what to aim for.

Age Group	Target Hold (Eyes Open)
20–49 years	30–60 seconds
50–59 years	20–40 seconds
60–69 years	10–30 seconds
70–79 years	5–20 seconds
80+ years	< 10 seconds

Why this matters for longevity: Studies have shown that adults unable to hold a single-leg stance for at least 10 seconds have a significantly higher risk of falls and all-cause mortality.[57] Improving your time even by a few seconds can make a meaningful difference to your long-term health.

Eyes-closed version: Once you can confidently balance for 30 seconds or more with your eyes open, test yourself with your eyes closed:

- Use the same form but close your eyes as soon as you lift your foot.
- This version is much harder.
- Most people can initially manage 2–5 seconds.
- Goal: aim to build up to 15 seconds per leg with practice.

As you progress through the plan, repeat this test every 7 days. Even minor improvements indicate a positive shift in your balance, stability and coordination, key factors in maintaining longevity and independence.

Write down your times for each leg and whether your eyes were open or closed. You'll be amazed at how quickly your nervous system adapts and improves.

2. Sit-to-Stand Test (30-Second Chair Stand Test)

Why are we testing this? This functional movement test assesses lower body strength, muscular endurance and your ability to perform everyday activities like standing from sitting on a loo, getting out of bed or climbing stairs. These are essential movements we often take for granted until they become difficult.

As we age, we naturally lose muscle mass, especially in the lower body. This loss, known as sarcopenia, can lead to frailty, increased fall risk and reduced independence. The Sit-to-Stand Test provides a quick yet powerful insight into the condition of your legs and whether your current strength is sufficient to support healthy ageing. Research indicates that lower body strength is one of the strongest predictors of functional independence as individuals age.[58] This test is one of the simplest and most effective ways to measure it.

How to do it:
1. Use a firm, armless, standard-height chair (about 43–45cm/17 inches high).
2. Sit upright, feet flat on the floor, hip-width apart.
3. Cross your arms over your chest so you're not using your hands to help.
4. On Go, stand up fully and sit back down as many times as possible within 30 seconds.
5. Make sure to stand up (hips and knees extended) and sit down fully each time.

6. Count your repetitions out loud or use a timer app with a counter.
7. Stop when 30 seconds is up.

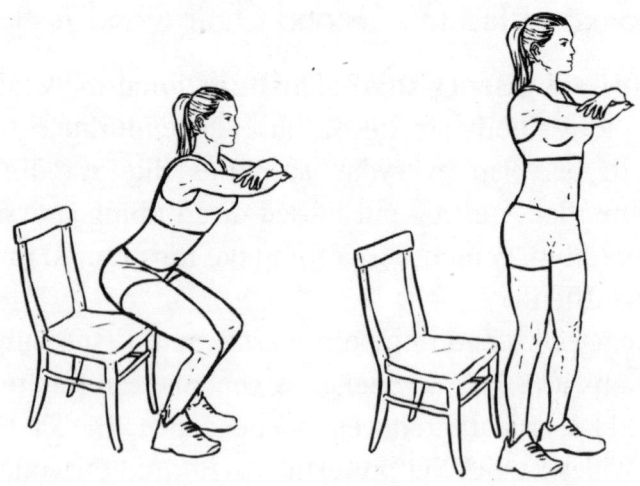

If you wobble or the form slips a bit during your last few reps, that's okay. This is about effort and capacity.

Goals and benchmarks: Use the benchmarks below to gauge your result. These figures are based on normative data for women and give a rough guide for what to aim for.

Age Group	Target Reps in 30 Seconds
40–49 years	→ 13 or more
50–54 years	→ 12 or more
55–64 years	→ 11 or more
65–69 years	→ 10 or more
70–79 years	→ 9 or more
80–84 years	→ 8 or more
85+	→ 7 or more

Fewer than 8 reps at any age may indicate a higher risk of falls, mobility limitations or reduced leg strength. However, remember that this is a starting point, not a final sentence. With consistent strength training, your number can and will improve.

Why this matters for longevity: Being able to repeatedly stand from a chair without using your arms signals that your quads, glutes, hamstrings and core are strong enough to support your weight, stabilise your spine and keep you moving well. Improved scores often translate to:

- Reduced fall risk
- Better walking speed and stability
- Lower risk of hospitalisation
- Greater independence in later life

Use this test not just to check progress but as part of your training. Regularly practising bodyweight sit-to-stands improves leg strength, heart rate response and overall confidence in movement.

Write down your reps every 7 days as per the programme.

3. Timed Up and Go (TUG) Test

Why are we testing this? The Timed Up and Go (TUG) test is a versatile tool for assessing mobility, walking speed, agility and balance, all of which are crucial for maintaining independence and confidence in daily life.

It replicates real-world movements: getting up from a chair, walking, turning and sitting back down. These are movements we perform dozens of times a day, often without thinking.

However, as we age, subtle changes in our movement can signal early declines in strength, coordination or reaction time, often before we notice them ourselves.

TUG is also a great indicator of brain-body coordination, especially relevant as we age and need to stay sharp both mentally and physically.

How to do it:
1. Use a standard-height chair with a firm seat and back support. Place it on a flat surface.
2. Sit in the chair with your back against the backrest, feet flat on the floor, arms resting in your lap.
3. On Go, stand up, walk 3 metres (10 feet) at a comfortable but brisk pace, turn around, walk back and sit down again.
4. Use a stopwatch or phone timer to measure the time from the moment you start moving to the moment you're fully seated again.
5. Perform the test at your normal walking pace, not a race – this is about efficiency and fluidity, not sprinting. Make sure the walking path is clear and safe.

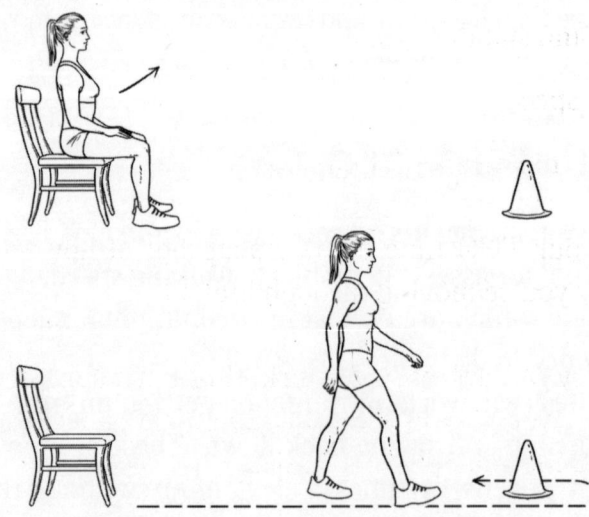

Goals and benchmarks: These time ranges are based on standard guidelines for what adults over 40 should be able to achieve and will help you understand your current level of functional mobility.

Age Group	Target TUG Time
40–49 years	→ 6 seconds or less
50–59 years	→ 7 seconds or less
60–69 years	→ 8 seconds or less
70–79 years	→ 9 seconds or less
80–89 years	→ 10 seconds or less
90+	→ 12 seconds or less

Why this matters for longevity: The TUG test reflects how well your body and brain work together to perform essential tasks. Completing this movement efficiently shows strong:

- lower body strength
- coordination
- balance and stability
- reaction speed
- cognitive-motor integration

In short, your TUG time offers a snapshot of how safely and confidently you're moving through life.

Retest every 7 days as you work through your plan. With consistency, you should see your time drop or feel the movement becoming smoother and easier.

4. Functional Reach Test

Why are we testing this? The Functional Reach Test assesses your dynamic balance and your ability to stay stable while your centre of gravity shifts forward. It's a practical, evidence-based method for measuring core and trunk stability, as well as fall risk.

We often reach forward in daily life, such as picking something up off the floor, reaching in a cupboard or grabbing a handrail. If your balance isn't strong, these slight movements can become risky. This test assesses your ability to move confidently and safely through space without overbalancing or stepping.

A strong performance in this test reflects solid core control, postural alignment and muscle coordination, all critical for preventing falls and maintaining long-term mobility.

How to do it:
1. Stand side-on next to a wall (non-dominant shoulder facing the wall).
2. Use a measuring tape or metre ruler affixed to the wall at shoulder height.
3. Extend your dominant arm straight forward, parallel to the floor, fingers outstretched. This is your starting position.
4. Reach forward as far as you can without taking a step, twisting your hips or losing balance. Keep your arm lifted and body stable.
5. Measure the distance from the start point (where your knuckles were at rest) to the furthest point reached while maintaining balance.
6. Record the distance in centimetres or inches.

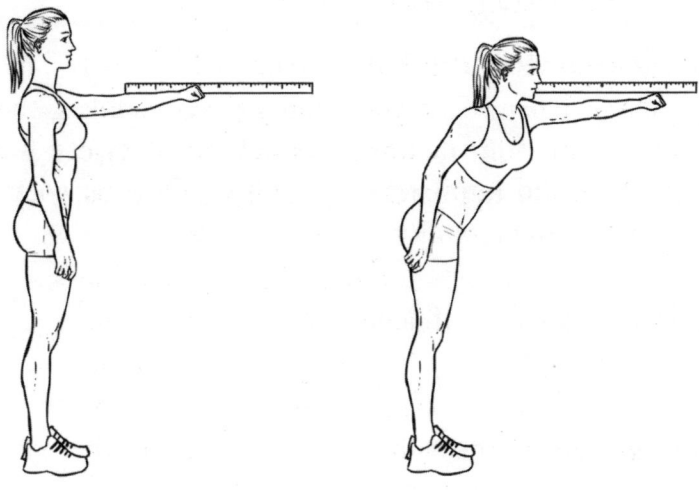

Tip: Keep your feet flat and planted. If you wobble or have to step, the test is invalid. It's all about how far you can reach while staying rooted.

Goals and benchmarks:

Reach Distance	Interpretation
25cm (10+ inches)	Excellent: good balance and trunk control
15–24cm (6–9½ inches)	Mild balance limitations
Under 15cm (6 inches)	Increased fall risk: needs improvement

Studies have found that a reach of less than 15cm (6 inches) is associated with a significantly increased risk of falls in older adults.

Why this matters for longevity: This test provides valuable insight into how well your core muscles, nervous system and balance mechanisms work together. A substantial functional reach shows that you can move confidently and maintain stability even when your body shifts outside its base of support.

It also indirectly reflects posture, shoulder mobility, spinal alignment and reaction time, making it one of the most comprehensive fall risk assessments available.

You can use this test regularly throughout your plan to track your progress and improvement. As you work on your core, glutes, balance and mobility, you'll likely notice:

- a smoother, more confident reach
- a longer distance without instability
- better posture and coordination

Retest every 7 days as you work through your plan. Even a few centimetres of extra reach can indicate meaningful improvement in trunk control and balance.

5. Press-Up Test (Modified or Standard)

Why are we testing this? This test assesses upper body strength and muscular endurance, specifically in the chest, shoulders, triceps and core. Strong upper body muscles aren't just about aesthetics, they're vital for daily tasks like lifting, pushing, carrying shopping or getting up from the floor.

Upper body strength is also linked to cardiovascular health, bone density and overall physical resilience, especially in midlife and beyond. Being able to perform a press-up well is a fantastic sign of functional fitness and muscle integrity.

Research has found that upper body strength (including press-up capacity) is linked to a lower risk of heart disease and premature death.[59]

How to do it:
Wall Press-Up (beginner)
- Stand facing a wall, arms extended, hands shoulder-width apart.
- Bend your elbows to bring your chest towards the wall, then push back to standing.

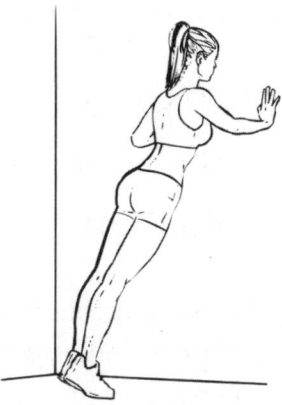

Modified Press-Up (beginner–intermediate)
- Start on your knees, hands slightly wider than shoulder-width apart.
- Keep a straight line from your shoulders to your knees.
- Lower your chest towards the floor (about a fist's width above) and press back up.

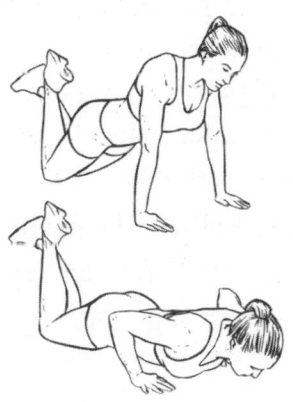

Standard Press-Up (advanced)

- Start on your toes, in a high plank.

- Engage your core and glutes to keep your body in one line.

- Lower down to just above the ground and push back up with control.

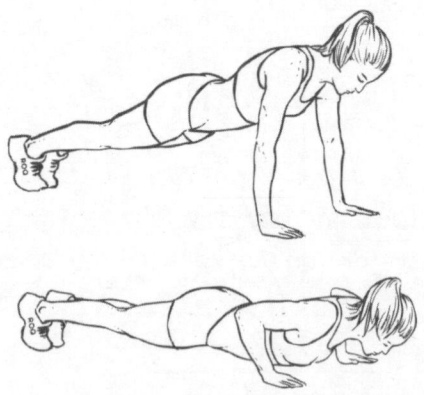

No matter the version, the key is good form: no sagging hips, flared elbows or half reps. Quality over quantity.

Goals and benchmarks:

Age 50+ (Women)	Interpretation
20+ modified press-ups	Excellent: strong and resilient
10–15 modified press-ups	Good upper body strength and endurance
< 10 press-ups	Improvement needed: work on strength

For those doing standard press-ups, scoring even 5–10 reps with good form is excellent.

Why this matters for longevity: Upper body strength is often overlooked, but it's crucial for independence, posture, joint protection and injury prevention, especially as we age. The ability to push yourself off the floor, hold your body weight and maintain strong posture is central to your quality of life in later years.

Test yourself every 3–4 weeks. If you're consistently training (even just once or twice a week), you'll likely notice:

- more reps
- better form
- greater ease with each attempt

Progress tip: Record the number of reps, the version used (wall, knees or toes) and how you felt after each rep. This can be a powerful motivator and confidence boost over time.

6. Squat Test

Why are we testing this? Squats are one of the most functional movements we can do. They mimic everyday actions like sitting down, standing up, bending to lift something and climbing stairs.

This test measures lower body strength, endurance, mobility and joint health. Strong legs help you move well, avoid falls and stay independent for longer. Leg strength has been shown to predict longevity, especially in women over 50.

It also helps highlight any issues with hip mobility, knee tracking or core stability, which may affect your posture and movement patterns.

If you want to stay mobile and confident as you age, building and maintaining leg strength is non-negotiable.

How to do it:
1. Stand with feet shoulder-width apart, toes slightly turned out.

2. Extend your arms out in front for balance if needed.
3. Begin your timer (30 seconds).
4. Lower into a squat by bending your hips and knees, keeping your chest lifted and knees tracking over your toes.
5. Go as deep as is comfortable, ideally to parallel or just above.
6. Return to standing and repeat as many times as possible in the time given.
7. Count only full squats with controlled movement and good form.

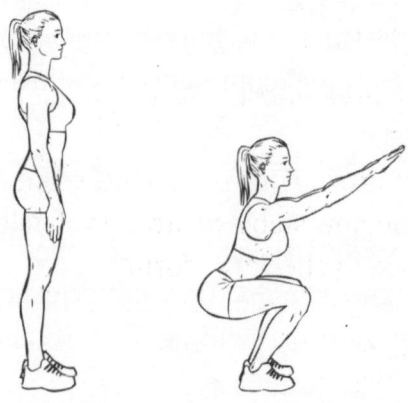

Don't rush. Focus on form over speed. Avoid letting your knees cave in or your heels lift off the ground.

Goals and benchmarks:

Age Group	Target Reps in 30 Seconds
40–49 years	15–17
50–59 years	12–14
60+ years	9–11

If you struggle to reach the recommended amount in 30 seconds or feel unstable, it's a sign to work on mobility, strength and coordination.

Why this matters for longevity: Leg strength helps you get up and down with ease, maintain better posture and move without fear of falling. It's also vital for maintaining a healthy metabolism and joint health. Squats activate the largest muscles in your body, making them one of the most efficient ways to build strength and functional fitness.

Retest every week. Over time, you'll likely notice:

- more reps
- smoother movement
- better squat depth
- less knee or hip discomfort

Progress tip: Jot down your rep count, squat depth ('parallel' or 'just above') and how stable or strong you felt during the test. Use video if needed to check the form.

7. 1-Mile Walk Test

Why are we testing this? This test measures cardiovascular endurance and aerobic fitness – two of the strongest indicators of heart health, metabolic function and overall longevity.

A brisk mile walk reflects how efficiently your heart, lungs and muscles work together. It's simple, accessible and backed by research as a powerful predictor of long-term health outcomes.

Studies show that better aerobic fitness is linked to lower risk of chronic diseases, improved cognitive function and a longer, healthier life, especially as we move through midlife and beyond.

How to do it:
1. Choose a flat, measured distance (1 mile = 1.6 km), such as a walking track, treadmill or a mapped route using a GPS app.
2. Warm up for a few minutes with gentle walking.
3. Start your timer and walk 1 mile as briskly as you can sustain – you should be working, but still able to speak.
4. Stop the timer when you finish.
5. (Optional) Measure your heart rate immediately at the end using a fitness tracker or by counting your pulse. Your pulse is your heart rate, or how many times your heart beats in a minute. To measure it, place two fingers (not your thumb) on your wrist or the side of your neck until you feel the beat. Count the beats for 30 seconds and double it, or for 60 seconds for accuracy.
6. Record your total time and, if possible, heart rate.

This is a walk, not a jog or run. You're aiming for your fastest *brisk walk* pace, not all-out effort.

Goals and benchmarks:

Age Group	Fair Time and Heart Rate	Target Time and Heart Rate
40s–50s	15–17 minutes/Heart rate more than 130 BPM	Less than 15 minutes/Heart rate less than 130 BPM
60s	15½–17½ minutes	Less than 15½ minutes/Heart rate less than 135 BPM
70s	16–18 minutes	Less than 16 minutes/Heart rate less than 140 BPM
80s	16½–18½ minutes	Less than 16½ minutes/Heart rate less than 145 BPM
90s	17–19 minutes	Less than 17 minutes/Heart rate less than 150 BPM

Faster time + lower heart rate at the end = better aerobic efficiency and heart health.

If your time is higher than these ranges or your heart rate spikes significantly, that may indicate reduced cardiovascular fitness. The good news? Endurance is highly trainable; even walking 2–3 times a week can make a huge difference.

Why this matters for longevity: The 1-Mile Walk Test reflects:

- heart strength and efficiency
- lung capacity
- circulation
- energy system resilience

Better cardiovascular fitness means more energy, reduced disease risk, better sleep, improved mood and increased chances of healthy ageing.

Test yourself every 7 days during the programme and record:

- time to complete the mile
- (optional) heart rate at the end
- how you felt (effort level, breathing, recovery)

Aim to walk the same route each time, under similar conditions (weather, surface, etc.), for consistent comparison.

The 7 Longevity Fitness Tests: What They Measure and Why They Matter

Test	What It Measures	Why It Matters
1. Single Leg Stand Test	Balance and proprioception	Predicts fall risk and overall longevity; supports coordination and ankle stability
2. Sit-to-Stand Test	Lower body strength and muscular endurance	Indicates ability to perform everyday tasks; linked to independence and fall risk
3. Timed Up and Go (TUG)	Agility, walking speed and balance	Reflects mobility, functional movement and brain–body coordination
4. Functional Reach Test	Dynamic balance and core/trunk stability	Highlights fall risk and postural control during real-world reaching movements
5. Press-Up Test	Upper body strength and endurance	Linked to cardiovascular health, posture and the ability to perform daily activities
6. Squat Test	Lower body strength, mobility and joint health	Assesses leg power, joint integrity and functional independence
7. 1-Mile Walk Test	Cardiovascular endurance and aerobic fitness	Strong predictor of heart health, metabolic function and longevity

Log Your Progress Throughout the 21-Day Plan in This Table

Test	Day 7	Day 14	Day 21	Day 28
1. Single Leg Stand Test (seconds)				
2. Sit-to-Stand Test (reps in 30 seconds)				
3. Timed Up and Go (seconds)				
4. Functional Reach Test (cm/inches)				
5. Press-Up Test (reps in 30 seconds)				
6. Squat Test (reps in 30 seconds)				
7. 1-Mile Walk (minutes and heart rate)				

PART 4
The 21-Day Plan

This is the part where you say yes to yourself. You're here for a reason, and I'm guessing it's because something inside you is ready for change. Not a quick fix, but something lasting. Something rooted in how you want to feel in your body, in your mind and in your life moving forwards.

This 21-Day Plan has been carefully designed to help you build sustainable habits that support strength, energy and clarity not just for today, but for years to come. It's not about overhauling your life overnight or chasing perfection. It's about taking consistent, manageable steps each day that compound into lasting change.

Each day follows the same structure – combining movement and mindset – because true longevity isn't just about how strong your body is, but also how steady your mind is and how supported you feel emotionally.

Here's what you can expect every day:

Warm-Up: 3–5 minutes of mobility

These short, purposeful warm-ups are designed to gently open up your joints, improve circulation and help you connect with your body before you start the main workout. Especially as we age, mobility is just as important as strength; it keeps us moving freely and confidently in daily life.

Main Sequence: 25 minutes of targeted movement

This is the core of your physical practice. Each sequence is focused on building functional strength, stability and endurance. You don't need a gym, expensive equipment or hours of free time, just your body, a bit of space and a willingness to show up. These 25 minutes are efficient but effective, and they're tailored for real midlife bodies navigating hormonal shifts, energy changes and busy lives.

Cool Down: 3-5 minutes

Cooling down is a vital part of every workout, especially when we're training for longevity. It helps the body transition from effort to rest, gradually lowering the heart rate and preventing dizziness or stiffness. More importantly, it supports recovery by improving circulation, reducing muscle soreness and calming the nervous system. In *The Longevity Solution,* these cool-down exercises aren't just about the cool down but also help with mobility and flexibility. It's about making sure your cool down becomes a habit

Journal Prompt: 5 minutes of reflection

Movement alone isn't enough. To create real, meaningful change, I've learnt that we also need to check in with our thoughts and emotions. Each day, I'll encourage you to journal, using simple prompts to help you reflect on what you're learning, how you're feeling and what habits are working for you.

Over the next 21 days, you'll start to notice changes, not just in how you move, but in how you think, how you feel and how you show up for your life. These aren't quick fixes. They're foundations. And every time you complete a day, you're laying another brick in your stronger, more resilient future.

You can follow the plan through the QR code below, which brings each session to life in real time. I'll be right there with you, guiding you through. And if you'd rather work from the book, everything you need is here on the following pages. You can also gain access to the Owning Your Menopause membership, where you can continue building strength for longevity after you finish your 21-day plan – use the code LONGEVITY50 for 50% off the first three months of membership.

Some of you might feel this isn't as intense as what you're used to, and that's okay. You're not doing less, you're doing differently. You're paying attention to what your body and mind need. You're filling in the gaps that get missed when we're stuck in autopilot. And for others, this might feel like a challenge. That's okay too. The goal isn't perfection. It's building strong, smart foundations that will support you through this chapter of life and the next.

Movement, mindset, journalling and nourishment all belong together. When they align, something shifts. You don't just feel stronger. You feel more yourself. More connected. More alive.

Each morning, you will warm up with the same mobility and warm-up drills, as I want you to consistently incorporate this routine. Repeating this routine will become a habit, something you keep for yourself and do three to four times a week after the end of the 21-Day Plan.

Disclaimer

Please review the following before starting the 21-Day Plan.

Note that this programme and the on-demand workouts have been designed to improve basic levels of fitness. It has not been designed for any specific issues that may be exacerbated by some of the more intense exercises.

Kate Rowe-Ham strongly recommends that you consult with your GP before beginning any exercise programme if you feel you have any pre-existing conditions. If you experience faintness, dizziness, pain or shortness of breath at any time while exercising, you should stop immediately. When participating in any exercise, there may be a possibility of physical injury. If you engage in the 21-Day Plan, then you agree that you do so at your own risk, are voluntarily participating in these activities, assume all risk of injury to yourself, and agree to release and discharge Kate Rowe-Ham from any claims. This programme offers health, fitness, nutritional and menopause information and is designed for educational purposes only. You should not rely on this information as a substitute for professional medical advice. The use of any information provided is at your own risk.

CHAPTER 26

Set Yourself up for Success

Right, let's be honest, we've all had that moment where we start a plan full of good intentions, only to find ourselves midweek wondering, 'What am I doing again?' So, let's take the guesswork out and really set ourselves up for success this time.

Here's how to go into your 21-Day Plan feeling prepared, confident and excited, not stressed and scrambling.

What you need to start

- **Equipment**

Please ensure you have a set of dumbbells, ideally 3kg and 5kg, as we will use these in the plan. This plan encourages you to get more mobile and stronger, and we want you to feel challenged.

- **A mat**

This will help protect your back when we do some of the abdominal exercises and provide a good base for stability. Carpets and wooden floors can be too slippery and could lead to injury.

- **A water bottle**

It is important to stay hydrated throughout your sessions. Ensure you have enough water to hand so your workout isn't interrupted.

- **Comfortable clothes to work out in**

These are essential. You don't need gym kit, you just need something light and comfortable.

- **Trainers**

I train barefoot to ensure my feet are grounded and stable. This can also strengthen your core, which helps increase balance. However, you can wear trainers – this is a matter of personal preference.

Know your 'Why'

Before you even think about movement or meals, take a moment to connect with why you're doing this.

Is it because you're fed up with feeling tired? Wanting to feel stronger? Keen to look after your future self? Write it down. Stick it on the fridge. Say it out loud. Your why is what you'll come back to on the days you can't be bothered.

Get real about your food

Let's talk meal prep, but not in the spend six hours cooking chicken and broccoli way. More like:

- Use the meal plan and guide provided and stick to it.

- Use the shopping list and get in what you need.

- Do a bit of batch prep: chop some veggies, cook a grain or two, boil some eggs, roast a tray of veg.

Think of it like laying the tracks so you're not derailed by a midweek panic about what to eat, which is when you often find yourself picking at things you don't need.

Plan your movement

If it's not in the diary, chances are it won't happen. I've created the 21-Day Plan for you – all I need is for you to follow along:

- Look at your week ahead and block out when you'll move – book it in like a meeting.
- Lay your kit out the night before if you're exercising in the morning.
- Know what you're doing – don't leave it to the last moment. Have your workout ready to go. Consistency beats intensity every time.

Tell people you're doing this

Seriously, don't keep it quiet. Tell your partner, your best friend, your WhatsApp group, even your Instagram followers if you're feeling brave. When you say it out loud, it becomes real and you're far more likely to stick with it.

Set yourself up physically and mentally.

The little things make a big difference:

- Water bottle filled.
- Healthy snacks prepped.

- Your favourite playlist ready.

- Even a sticky note that says, 'You've got this' on the mirror.

Use the journal

Whether it's ticking a box or jotting a sentence in the daily journal, please track your days. Not to be obsessive, but to reflect. 'How did that feel?' 'What helped me today?' 'What made it harder?' This builds self-awareness, and that's what really changes the game long term.

Commit. Properly.
 Commit like you mean it.
 Not, 'I'll try and see how I go.' Nope. It's, 'I'm doing this for 21 Days. I owe it to myself.'

CHAPTER 27

Why the Exercises in This Plan Work for Longevity

We've established by now that as we move through midlife, our goals around exercise often shift. It's no longer just about chasing aesthetic goals, shrinking our bodies or squeezing into a smaller dress size. Instead, it becomes about how we feel in our bodies, how we move, how we stand, how we show up in our everyday lives.

It's about moving with ease, reducing stiffness, staying strong and balanced, and having the energy and resilience to do the things we love without pain, strain or hesitation. It's about knowing that the way we move today is laying the foundations for a vibrant, independent future.

That's precisely why I created this plan: to help you reconnect with your body, rebuild your strength and feel empowered through movement no matter your starting point.

Every exercise you'll find here has been intentionally chosen with longevity in mind. The focus is not on flashy workouts or complicated routines, but on functional movements that support you in real life today, tomorrow and ten years from now. These are the patterns that help you pick up your shopping bags without straining your back; get up off the floor with ease; twist, reach, bend and balance without hesitation or fear of falling.

The daily sessions are rooted in three key principles: strength, mobility and balance. Together, they form the foundation for ageing well. This isn't about training harder; it's about training smarter. That's why the plan starts with bodyweight and low-resistance options. Form matters more than load. And if you're just getting started, body weight can be more than enough to spark change. You'll build neuromuscular coordination, reconnect with muscles that may have been asleep for years, and relearn how to move well, something that gets overlooked all too easily in midlife.

Muscle Imbalance

Have you ever noticed that one side of your body feels stronger? This could be a sign of muscle imbalance. It is not uncommon to have muscular imbalances from carrying out day-to-day activities, such as picking up children and carrying them on one side, or from sitting at home, in the car or at work.

Indicators include uneven balance or flexibility in your body. Poor posture is a cause and symptom of muscle imbalance, which can occur when you sit for long periods or maintain incorrect posture when standing or sitting. Over time, this can leave specific muscles underworked and weak.

Regular workouts or exercise help strengthen most muscle groups. Unilateral training will be beneficial in addressing these imbalances. It is incorporated into the 21-Day Plan because it is an integral part of becoming fitter and stronger and can be a key in injury prevention too, preventing overtraining of the dominant side and correcting imbalances.

Treatment for severe muscle imbalance will vary, and if you feel this could be you, please seek specific help from a specialist.

Why Add Weights?

Here's the key: as you get stronger, you must challenge the body in new ways. That's where weights come in. Lifting heavier isn't about pushing beyond your limits, it's about giving your body the resistance it needs to adapt and thrive. Our muscles need stress to grow; our bones need impact to stay strong. Especially in a postmenopausal body, where hormonal shifts naturally accelerate the loss of both muscle mass and bone density, adding external load becomes not just helpful but essential.

You can start with 3kg dumbbells, or even lighter. As your confidence grows, so will your capacity to handle more. A few weeks later, 5kg might feel just right. Eventually, 8kg becomes your new normal. This progression doesn't need to be forced. It will happen naturally if you stick with the process, listen to your body and trust the plan.

One of the most powerful aspects of the 21-Day Plan is that it's designed to be repeated. You don't need a new workout every week to progress. Repeating this plan will give you the consistency required for real change. The first time through, it might feel like a steep learning curve. You'll be focused on simply getting through it, learning the movements, understanding your breath and tuning into your form. That's enough.

When you return to it, because you will want to, you'll notice you can move with more control. You might hold a position longer, slow the tempo and add resistance. That's progression. It's not always about adding more weight or reps. Sometimes it's about adding more intention. And that intention is what rewires your body and your mindset for lasting strength.

Another way of progressing is to slow down the lowering phase of each movement; this way you increase time under tension. You could try this if your weights don't feel heavy enough. This simple tweak challenges the muscles in a completely different way and enables even greater adaptation. It teaches you patience, precision and power, not just physically but mentally too.

So, don't rush to the next programme. This plan is designed to meet you where you are and to grow with you. It is your anchor: a consistent, flexible, repeatable foundation that you can return to again and again. In a world that constantly tells us to do more, lift more, move faster, this is your permission to slow down, get intentional and train in a way that supports your body for life.

You don't need to train for punishment or performance. You're training for the possibility of all the things you still want to do in the years to come.

> ### The Importance of Warming Up
> The 21-Day Plan is not just about getting a workout done, it's also about how we prepare for the session to prevent injury. This forms an integral part of the plan because even if you have a good fitness level, many people forget to warm up and cool down, which can impact recovery. Simply adding these two key components can be transformative.
>
> As we age, our joints naturally lose mobility, our muscles tighten and our connective tissues become less elastic. Without regular stretching and mobility work, this can lead to stiffness, reduced range of motion, poor posture and an increased risk of injury, not just during workouts but in everyday life. Think: struggling to reach down, turn your head when driving or even get up from the floor.
>
> Here's why I've chosen each of these specific exercises for the warm-up:

- **Bent Knee Calf Stretch and Downward Dog Knee Bend:** These movements target the calves and Achilles, which are often tight and can impact gait, ankle mobility and balance. Improving flexibility here supports better walking, squatting and running mechanics.
- **Ankle Circles:** Mobility at the ankle is crucial for balance and reducing fall risk. These simple circles lubricate the joint and improve proprioception, the body's ability to sense where it is in space.
- **Good Morning!:** This is a great way to wake up the posterior chain hamstrings, glutes and lower back. It encourages hip hinge mechanics, vital for protecting your back during everyday movements like bending or lifting.
- **World's Greatest Stretch:** A big, dynamic stretch that hits almost everything: hips, hamstrings, thoracic spine and shoulders. It's ideal for opening up the body before movement and improving full-body mobility.
- **Thread the Needle:** Many people's mid-backs are tight due to their sedentary lifestyles. This stretch improves rotation through the spine, which is essential for everything from reaching across the body to turning while driving.
- **Walkout (to knees if needed):** This move activates the core, stretches the posterior chain and builds functional upper-body strength. It also mimics the movements that are required for getting up and down from the floor – an essential longevity marker.

Don't skip the warm-up (see page 240), especially if you want to make the most of this plan.

The Importance of Cooling Down

What we do after exercise is just as important as before, especially for long-term health and mobility. Cooling down and stretching after a workout helps our body transition from high intensity to rest.

Cool-down stretches help gradually slow the heart rate, reduce post-exercise soreness, promote circulation and calm the nervous system. They also provide a moment of stillness, giving the body and mind space to recover. Here's why these specific movements matter so much and form part of the cool-down in the plan:

- **Child's Pose:** This gentle stretch calms the nervous system and lengthens the spine, hips and lower back. It's a grounding position that helps release tension in key areas affected by daily posture and stress.
- **Happy Baby Pose:** Ideal for opening the hips and stretching the lower back, this pose gently targets the inner thighs and groin. Hip mobility is vital for balance, walking and preventing lower back strain as we age.
- **Cobra:** A brilliant chest-opener that counters all the forward-hunched positions we spend time in. It also strengthens the lower back, promotes spinal extension and helps with posture, which is essential for maintaining a tall, confident stance as we age.
- **Cat Cows:** This gentle spinal movement improves flexibility and control throughout the back. It's a great way to ease stiffness, reduce tension and maintain a healthy, mobile spine.
- **Thoracic Rotation:** This is vital for maintaining mobility in the upper and mid-back. It supports posture, balance and breathing and helps offset the effects of a sedentary lifestyle and poor desk posture.

Making these stretches part of your cool-down routine (see page 240) doesn't just feel good in the moment; it will protect your body in the long run. They help maintain joint integrity, prevent muscular imbalances and promote overall flexibility, which means more ease and freedom in everything from getting dressed to reaching overhead or playing with grandchildren.

CHAPTER 28

Journalling for the 21-Day Plan

In Chapter 20, I discussed the different types of journalling, their benefits and the numerous advantages they offer. I know how alien this practice might be for many of you and I was once very sceptical too, but I would like to invite you over the next 21 days to give it a try.

With your daily journal, I encourage you to have a morning and evening check-in, focusing on your physical and mental state, and also record what you did so you can see how this has impacted your physical, emotional and mental well-being. This daily journal is a Health and Habit Journal (see page 167).

You can expand on the Weekly Check-In and go in any direction you like. It can be more detailed if you carve out some time or you could try some of the other forms of journalling to see how that feels (see pages 162–169).

Your Daily Journal

This daily journal is designed to support your progress over the 21 days – physically, emotionally and mentally. Each page prompts you to reflect, notice how your body feels and stay anchored in the small daily actions that lead to lasting change.

You don't have to write long entries, just enough to check in with yourself and honour the effort you're making.

Morning Check-In
How do I feel this morning?
(energised, tired, motivated, anxious, calm, etc.)
My intention for today:
(move more, eat well, be kind to myself, etc.)

Movement
☐ **Day [ ] completed**

Extras *(tick any that apply)*:
☐ Strength training
☐ Walk outdoors
☐ Other: _____

Nutrition
Meals today: *(note key nutrients or highlights)*

- **Breakfast:** _____
- **Lunch:** _____
- **Dinner:** _____
- **Snacks:** _____

Water intake: _____ glasses *(aim for 6–8)*

Food Focus

Did I include...
- ☐ A source of protein in each meal?
- ☐ Colourful fruit or vegetables today?
- ☐ Whole, minimally processed foods?

How did eating today make me feel?
(satisfied, bloated, energised, sluggish, etc.)

Mindful Moment

Did I take a moment to pause and breathe today?
☐ Yes ☐ No
Did I do something enjoyable or relaxing?
☐ Yes ☐ No
Did I connect with a friend or loved one?
☐ Yes ☐ No

Evening Reflection

One positive moment today:
_____

What could I improve tomorrow (gently)?
_____

Gratitude – one thing I'm grateful for:
_____

Your Weekly Check-In (Every 7 Days)

Take a few extra moments at the end of each week to notice how you're evolving. Write freely and honestly; this is for you.

What habit am I most proud of sticking with?
_____

What's becoming easier or more natural?
_____

One small tweak to improve next week:
_____

CHAPTER 29

Alongside the Plan, Some Simple Exercise Hacks for Longevity

While the plan will help you achieve gains in mobility, balance and strength – all of which will positively impact future health outcomes – realistically, we need to ensure that we don't rely solely on this approach. All daily movement will contribute to your overall well-being, and the more you move, the better you'll feel. With that in mind, alongside the plan, I would love you to consider adding other ways to help you move, age better and live longer.

I've provided a few ideas here. Select one or two of these habits and incorporate them into your daily routine. The more you move with intention and consistency, the stronger, healthier and more resilient your body will become, regardless of age.

Get up every 30 minutes

The reality is that many of us sit far too much. Research has shown that sitting for more than 8 hours a day is linked to a 17–49% higher risk of early death, even for people who exercise regularly.[60] A sedentary lifestyle increases the risk of heart disease, obesity, diabetes and even cognitive decline. Set a reminder to stand up and move every 30–60 minutes. Even short bursts of movement, like stretching, walking around the house or doing bodyweight squats, can break up long periods of sitting and counteract its adverse effects.

Walk after meals

A 10–15-minute walk after eating has been shown to reduce blood sugar spikes by up to 30%, helping to lower the risk of type 2 diabetes and metabolic disorders.[61] Walking also improves digestion, reduces stress and enhances circulation, making it one of the easiest and most effective ways to boost overall well-being and longevity. Instead of sitting down after meals, go for a 10-minute walk, even if it's just around your home or office.

Leg strength

You might be surprised to learn that leg strength significantly predicts longevity. Strong legs improve balance, mobility and independence as we age. In contrast, weak legs heighten the risk of falls, leading to long-term health complications for older adults. Try adding 10–15 squats to your daily routine; do them while brushing your teeth, waiting for your coffee to brew or during TV commercial breaks.

Practise 1-minute balance holds

Good balance isn't just about preventing falls; it's directly linked to brain health and longevity. Studies have shown that poor balance can predict earlier mortality, particularly as we age. Practising a single-leg balance for just 1 minute on each leg daily can strengthen stabilising muscles, improve proprioception and stimulate the brain. Start by standing near a wall or chair for support. As you improve, try closing your eyes or turning your head slowly while balancing to challenge your coordination and improve your balance.

Carry something heavy (safely)

Loaded carries, such as farmer's carries (which are included in the plan), mimic real-life strength tasks and promote grip strength, posture and full-body endurance. Grip strength alone is a powerful predictor of lifespan. You don't need a gym: carry shopping bags evenly in both hands, use filled water bottles or repurpose household items. Walk slowly and intentionally for 30–60 seconds a few times a week. Focus on standing tall with your shoulders back and core engaged.

Daily breathwork

Breathing is something we all do, but how we breathe can have a profound impact on our stress levels, recovery and even longevity. Breathwork activates the parasympathetic nervous system (our rest and digest mode), helping to lower blood pressure, reduce inflammation, improve focus and aid recovery. Begin with a simple practice, such as Box Breathing (inhale for 4 seconds, hold for 4 seconds, exhale for 4 seconds, hold for 4 seconds), for just 2–5 minutes daily. Do it first thing in the morning, during a stressful moment or before bed to unwind. Try pairing your breathwork with movement. Breathe slowly during your cool-down session, stretch or even while walking.

CHAPTER 30

Let's Go

This is where your transformation starts. It's also something I encourage you to share. If you have a loved one – such as a partner, parent, sibling or friend – who could benefit from feeling stronger, more capable and more connected to their health, invite them to join you. Doing this together creates accountability, support and a shared sense of momentum. It's amazing how making positive changes in your own life can ripple out and lift the people around you, too.

I know that change can feel daunting, especially if you're still experiencing some of the more overwhelming symptoms of menopause, whether that's fatigue, anxiety or a general feeling of being disconnected from your body. But I hope that by now, through the pages of this book, you've begun to reconnect with what's possible. You've started to build trust in your ability to shift direction, to feel better and to take ownership of your well-being. You're not waiting for the right time, you're starting now, with what you have.

You don't need to carve out hours each day. Your movement routine will take no longer than 40 minutes, and it doesn't have to all be done together. Ideally that 40 minutes includes journalling, but I don't want you to feel pressured to limit yourself with this – take as much time as you need.

- **Warm-Up – Mobility and Balance (3–5 minutes):** Dynamic stretches and simple balance drills to wake up the body and reconnect with how it moves.

- **Main Sequence – Strength and Stability (25 minutes):** A short, effective sequence of bodyweight and resistance exercises designed to build muscular strength, joint integrity and postural awareness.

- **Cool-Down (3–5 minutes):** Simple stretches to calm the mind and ease the body.

- **Mindful Well-Being – Journalling (5 minutes):** A grounding practice to set your mental tone for the day, whether through breathwork or journalling.

If you haven't already, now's the time to start journalling. As part of this plan, I encourage you to commit to daily journalling and your weekly check-in, small but powerful tools to help you reflect, stay consistent and notice what's shifting, inside and out. Whether journalling is new to you or something you're returning to, this simple practice can make a big difference. Just jotting down a few bullet points each morning can help anchor your intentions and keep you focused.

Paired with the menu ideas you'll find in Part 5, this 21-Day Plan offers not just structure, but freedom, the kind that comes from knowing you're finally building something for yourself that lasts.

Let this be your starting line. And when you reach Day 21, come back to the plan. Repeat it. Adjust it. Invite someone else to join. The movements may stay the same, but *you* won't be.

You'll be stronger, more grounded and more aware of what your body is truly capable of.

> **A Day in the Life: Putting It All Into Practice**
> Here's how one day might look when you're fully embracing the 21-Day Plan and what most of my days look like. Movement, mindful nourishment and a moment to reset.
>
> ## Morning
> **Wake-Up Ritual (6:00 am)**
> I reach for the glass of water I leave by my bed and drink it. Head downstairs to the kitchen, and for me, it's my probiotic shot followed by coffee 10 minutes later. Before diving into the day, I pause for my Morning Check-In to ask myself: 'How do I want to feel today?' I take a moment to breathe, set an intention and get moving.
>
> **Movement: Daily Warm-Up + Main Sequence (6:30 am)**
> Today's plan:
> - **Warm-Up:** Ankle Circles, World's Greatest Stretch and Thread the Needle
> - **Main Sequence:** Lower body strength – Squats, Lunges, Hip Thrusts and Dead Bugs
> - **Cool-Down:** Child's Pose, Happy Baby Pose and Cobra
>
> I finish feeling grounded and strong, not drained, just energised.
> Get everyone ready for school, check emails and make my breakfast to eat on return from the school run.
>
> **Breakfast (9:15 am)**
> Protein-Packed Yoghurt Bowl

A reminder from my journal: 'I fuel my body to feel my best, not to punish or restrict.'

Midday
Lunch (1:30 pm)
Wholemeal wrap with hummus, grilled courgette, red pepper, rocket and a boiled egg
Side of edamame beans with a dash of sea salt
Herbal tea or a glass of still water

Mindful Moment (2:00 pm)
I step outside, go for a walk (if time), even just for 10 minutes.

Evening
Dinner (6:30 pm)
Lentil & Sweet Potato Burrito Mix
Small handful of mixed seeds sprinkled on top
Glass of water with cucumber and mint

Wind Down (8:00 pm)
No screens for the last 30 minutes.
For my Evening Reflection, I write down three things I'm grateful for and one win from the day, however small.
Tonight's evening reflection: 'What does tomorrow look like?' 'How can I improve?'

Weekly Check-In Tip: At the end of the week, I look back on my journal entries and highlight any patterns. Did my energy dip after poor sleep? Did my mood improve on strength training days? This helps me tune in and keep going, not perfectly, but consistently.

21 Days of Change

Days 1–7

In the first week, as you focus on form, mobility and control, you may begin to notice subtle but meaningful changes in how your body feels and moves. There's a growing awareness of imbalances or stiffness, and everyday actions like bending, reaching or getting up from the floor become smoother and more stable. By slowing down and prioritising quality over quantity, you'll engage the correct muscles more effectively, activating smaller stabilisers you might not usually feel, which can lead to new areas of soreness. Mobility work brings a sense of ease and freedom to your joints, while the deliberate pace sharpens your mind–muscle connection and helps reduce compensations or reliance on momentum. Perhaps most importantly, there's often a mental shift, as you begin to value moving well over simply moving more, creating a foundation for long-term strength and resilience.

Days 8–14

You may start to feel stronger, more stable and more connected to how your body moves. Having checked in with the tests and your progress on Day 7, you may have recorded which movements feel more fluid, where you have greater control, and where there's still room for improvement. With a solid foundation in form and mobility, you can begin to make it more challenging. You could slow down your tempo to increase time under tension or introduce light weights to build strength without compromising control. These subtle shifts encourage your body to adapt and grow stronger, while reinforcing proper movement patterns. You may find a renewed sense of focus, deeper core engagement, and a quiet confidence in your ability.

Days 15–21

You'll likely feel more confident in your movement patterns, with improved stability, coordination and strength. This final phase is about building on everything you've established, further progressing by increasing intensity in a controlled and purposeful way. You might add higher reps, incorporate combination moves that link strength with mobility or slightly increase load if your body feels ready. These progressions challenge your endurance, coordination and muscular control, helping to consolidate gains and push past earlier limits. By now, movement feels more intuitive, your posture and balance may be noticeably better, and you'll likely experience a stronger connection between effort and outcome, proof that consistency and intention truly drive transformation.

The Longevity Solution 21-Day Exercise Plan

DAY 1	DAY 2	DAY 3	DAY 4	DAY 5
Squats	Squats	Squats	Cat Cows	Squats
Press-Ups	Single-Arm Overhead Presses	Chest Presses	Bird Dog	Press-Ups
Good Morning!		Dumbbell	Thread the	Hip Thrusts
Reverse Lunges	Single-Leg	RDLs	Needle	Bent Arm
Twists	Thrusts	Side Lunges	Hip Flexors	Lateral
Suitcase Carry	Forward Lunges	Dead Bugs	Piriformis	Raises
(25 minutes)	(with chair)	Farmer's	Stretch	Overhead
	Plank Taps	Carry	Child's Pose	Presses
	Suitcase Carry	(25 minutes)	(20 minutes)	(25 minutes)
	(25 minutes)			

DAY 6	DAY 7	DAY 8	DAY 9	DAY 10
Squat Thrusters	REPEAT LONGEVITY TESTS	Squat Jumps or Squats	Split Squats	Cat Cows
Upright Rows		Push Presses	Chest Presses	Bird Dog
Mountain Climbers		Dumbbell RDLs	Single-Leg Thrusts	Thread the Needle
Curtsy Lunges		Reverse Lunges	Side Lunges	Hip Flexors
Dead Bugs		Crunch Taps	Press-Ups	Piriformis Stretch
(25 minutes)		Farmer's Carry	Bikes	Child's Pose
		(25 minutes)	(25 minutes)	(20 minutes)

DAY 11	DAY 12	DAY 13	DAY 14	DAY 15
Sumo Squats	REPEAT LONGEVITY TESTS	Slow Squats	Cat Cows	Squats
Bent-Over Row		Chest Presses	Bird Dog	Bent-Over Row
Reverse Lunges		Single-Leg RDL	Thread the Needle	Bent Arm Lateral Raises
Biceps		Side Lunges	Hip Flexors	
Upright Rows		Mountain Climbers	Piriformis Stretch	Reverse Lunges
Dead Bugs		Farmer's Carry	Child's Pose	Mountain Climbers
Overhead Presses		(25 minutes)	(20 minutes)	Farmer's Carry
(25 minutes)				(25 minutes)

DAY 16	DAY 17	DAY 18	DAY 19	DAY 20
Squats Press-Ups Hip Thrusts Reverse Lunges Biceps Bikes Suitcase Carry (25 minutes)	REPEAT LONGEVITY TESTS	Squat Thrusters Bent-Over Row Dumbbell RDLs Reverse Lunges Twists Suitcase Carry (25 minutes)	Cat Cows Bird Dog Thread the Needle Hip Flexors Piriformis Stretch Child's Pose (20 minutes)	Squats Chest Presses Plank Taps Side Lunges Twists Farmer's Carry (25 minutes)

DAY 21	FINAL TESTS
Squats Overhead Presses Reverse Lunges Biceps Dumbbell RDLs Twists Single-Leg Thrusts Farmer's Carry (30 minutes)	REPEAT LONGEVITY TESTS

Your Warm-Up and Cool-Down

Warm-Up Routine	Time / Reps
Bent Knee Calf Stretch Downward Dog Knee Bend	30–60 secs hold each side
Ankle Circles	10 circles each way, each ankle
Good Morning!	8 reps
World's Greatest Stretch	10 reps / 2–3 secs hold
Thread the Needle	3 reps each side / 2–3 secs hold
Walkouts (to knees if needed)	8 reps
	REPEAT x 2

Cool-Down Routine	Time / Reps
Child's Pose	15–30 secs hold
Happy Baby Pose	15–30 secs hold
Cobra	15 secs hold
Cat Cows	6 reps / 2–3 secs hold
Thoracic Rotation	15–30 secs hold
	REPEAT x 2

Day 1 We are starting with our Morning Check-In. How do you feel about getting started? Excited? Nervous? Today we are going to do some of the fundamental moves to include in your routines, which will ensure lifelong mobility and strength. Some of you may want to do this with chair support depending on your levels. Don't forget to start with your warm-up (page 240).

Exercises	Round 1	Round 2	Round 3
Squats (with chair) (page 266)	14 reps	12 reps	10 reps
Press-Ups (kneeling if needed (page 269)	14 reps	12 reps	10 reps
Good Morning! (page 259)	14 reps	12 reps	10 reps
Reverse Lunges (with chair) (page 275)	10 reps each side	8 reps each side	6 reps each side
Twists (page 285)	14 reps	12 reps	10 reps
Suitcase Carry (page 290)	Walk for 30–60 secs	Walk for 30–60 secs	Walk for 30–60 secs
	REST AFTER EACH ROUND FOR 45 SECS	REST AFTER EACH ROUND FOR 45 SECS	REST AFTER EACH ROUND FOR 45 SECS

Day 2 Another day of functional moves and mobility. I have included some unilateral work here as it is important to think about and work on any imbalances, especially when it comes to your balance and stability.

Exercises	Round 1	Round 2	Round 3
Squats (with chair) (page 266)	14 reps	12 reps	10 reps
Single-Arm Overhead Presses (page 281)	10 reps each side	8 reps each side	6 reps each side
Single-Leg Thrusts (page 280)	10 reps each side	10 reps each side	10 reps each side
Forward Lunges (with chair) (page 274)	10 reps each side	8 reps each side	6 reps each side
Plank Taps (page 283)	10 taps each side	10 taps each side	10 taps each side
Suitcase Carry (page 290)	Walk for 30–60 secs	Walk for 30–60 secs	Walk for 30–60 secs
	REST AFTER EACH ROUND FOR 45 SECS	REST AFTER EACH ROUND FOR 45 SECS	REST AFTER EACH ROUND FOR 45 SECS

Day 3 More functional moves, so that you can see over the last couple of days how training the body to move and mimic daily movement is key to longevity and living independently for as long as possible.

Exercises	Round 1	Round 2	Round 3
Squats (with chair) (page 266)	14 reps	12 reps	10 reps
Chest Presses (page 287)	14 reps	12 reps	10 reps
Dumbbell RDLs (page 273)	14 reps	12 reps	10 reps
Side Lunges (page 278)	10 reps each side	8 reps each side	6 reps each side
Dead Bugs (page 282)	10 reps each side	10 reps each side	10 reps each side
Farmer's Carry (page 289)	Walk for 30–60 secs	Walk for 30–60 secs	Walk for 30–60 secs
	REST AFTER EACH ROUND FOR 45 SECS	REST AFTER EACH ROUND FOR 45 SECS	REST AFTER EACH ROUND FOR 45 SECS

Day 4 Stretching away some possible aches from previous days. Please remember we are aiming for slow, sustainable change and progress.

Exercises	Round 1	Round 2	Round 3
Cat Cows (page 256)	8 reps	8 reps	8 reps
Bird Dog (page 259)	10 reps each side	10 reps each side	10 reps each side
Thread the Needle (page 257)	5 reps each side	5 reps each side	5 reps each side
Hip Flexors (page 260)	4 reps each side	4 reps each side	4 reps each side
Piriformis Stretch (page 261)	Hold 45 secs each side (count in your head if no timer)	Hold 45 secs each side (count in your head if no timer)	Hold 45 secs each side (count in your head if no timer)
Child's Pose (page 262)	30 secs	30 secs	30 secs
	REST AFTER EACH ROUND FOR 45 SECS	REST AFTER EACH ROUND FOR 45 SECS	REST AFTER EACH ROUND FOR 45 SECS

Day 5 Full-body moves here focusing on Upper and Lower with an excellent core finish. How is the body feeling after a gentler day yesterday? Has the rest allowed you to squat heavier or without support?

Exercises	Round 1	Round 2	Round 3
Squats (page 265)	14 reps	12 reps	10 reps
Press-Ups (page 269)	14 reps	12 reps	10 reps
Hip Thrusts (page 279)	15–30 secs x 5	15–30 secs x 5	15–30 secs x 5
Bent Arm Lateral Raises (page 272)	10 reps	8 reps	6 reps
Overhead Presses (page 280)	14 reps	12 reps	10 reps
	REST AFTER EACH ROUND FOR 45 SECS	REST AFTER EACH ROUND FOR 45 SECS	REST AFTER EACH ROUND FOR 45 SECS

Day 6 Before we head into testing on Day 7, I've added a couple more moves. The curtsy lunges work on moving laterally across a different plane, and then upright rows work on shoulder stability and strength.

Exercises	Round 1	Round 2	Round 3
Squat Thrusters (page 268)	14 reps	12 reps	10 reps
Upright Rows (page 271)	14 reps	12 reps	10 reps
Mountain Climbers (page 288)	10 reps each side	10 reps each side	10 reps each side
Curtsy Lunges (with chair) (page 276)	10 reps	8 reps	6 reps
Dead Bugs (page 282)	10 reps each side	10 reps each side	10 reps each side
	REST AFTER EACH ROUND FOR 45 SECS	REST AFTER EACH ROUND FOR 45 SECS	REST AFTER EACH ROUND FOR 45 SECS

Day 7 REPEAT LONGEVITY TESTS. This will be the first time repeating the tests and, hopefully, you may already notice some improvement on some of the exercises. If you don't, please don't worry. It takes time. Keep going, and I guarantee you will feel and see more benefits over the next 7 days.

Tests (page 190)	
Single Leg Stand	
Sit-to-Stand	
Timed Up and Go	
Functional Reach	
Press-Up	
Squat	
1-Mile Walk	

Day 8 Another full-body session focusing on building overall strength. For us to feel improvements, we are focusing on one muscle group per move, so that hopefully you can lift heavier weights in each round, if you feel ready.

Exercises	Round 1	Round 2	Round 3
Squat Jumps or Squats (with chair) (pages 267 and 266)	14 reps	12 reps	10 reps
Push Presses (page 287)	14 reps	12 reps	10 reps
Dumbbell RDLs (page 273)	14 reps	12 reps	10 reps
Reverse Lunges (page 275)	10 reps each side	8 reps each side	6 reps each side
Crunch Taps (page 284)	14 reps	12 reps	10 reps
Farmer's Carry (page 289)	Walk for 30–60 secs	Walk for 30–60 secs	Walk for 30–60 secs
	REST AFTER EACH ROUND FOR 45 SECS	REST AFTER EACH ROUND FOR 45 SECS	REST AFTER EACH ROUND FOR 45 SECS

Day 9 Another full-body session focusing on building all over strength with some of those unilateral moves we have done before.

Exercises	Round 1	Round 2	Round 3
Split Squats (with or without chair) (page 277)	8 reps each side	8 reps each side	8 reps each side
Chest Presses (page 287)	10 reps each side	8 reps each side	6 reps each side
Single-Leg Thrusts (page 280)	10 reps each side	10 reps each side	10 reps each side
Side Lunges (page 278)	10 reps each side	8 reps each side	6 reps each side
Press-Ups (page 269)	14 reps	12 reps	10 reps
Bikes (page 284)	10 each side	10 each side	10 each side
	REST AFTER EACH ROUND FOR 45 SECS	REST AFTER EACH ROUND FOR 45 SECS	REST AFTER EACH ROUND FOR 45 SECS

Day 10 Stretching away some possible aches from previous days. Please remember we are aiming for slow, sustainable change and progress.

Exercises	Round 1	Round 2	Round 3
Cat Cows (page 256)	8 reps	8 reps	8 reps
Bird Dog (page 259)	10 reps each side	10 reps each side	10 reps each side
Thread the Needle (page 257)	5 reps each side	5 reps each side	5 reps each side
Hip Flexors (page 260)	4 reps each side	4 reps each side	4 reps each side
Piriformis Stretch (page 261)	Hold 45 secs each side (count in your head if no timer)	Hold 45 secs each side (count in your head if no timer)	Hold 45 secs each side (count in your head if no timer)
Child's Pose (page 262)	30 secs	30 secs	30 secs
	REST AFTER EACH ROUND FOR 45 SECS	REST AFTER EACH ROUND FOR 45 SECS	REST AFTER EACH ROUND FOR 45 SECS

Day 11 Another opportunity to think about adding weights to some of these moves. This one will get the heart rate up.

Exercises	Round 1	Round 2	Round 3
Sumo Squats (page 267)	14 reps	12 reps	10 reps
Bent-Over Row (page 271)	10 reps each side	8 reps each side	6 reps each side
Reverse Lunges Biceps (page 276)	12 reps each side	10 reps each side	8 reps each side
Upright Rows (page 271)	10 reps	8 reps	6 reps
Dead Bugs (page 282)	10 reps each side	10 reps each side	10 reps each side
Overhead Presses (page 280)	12 reps	10 reps	8 reps
	REST AFTER EACH ROUND FOR 45 SECS	REST AFTER EACH ROUND FOR 45 SECS	REST AFTER EACH ROUND FOR 45 SECS

Day 12 REPEAT LONGEVITY TESTS. I'm excited for you to monitor and see what progress you have made. It may be small, but it is progress. Remember, Rome wasn't built in a day.

Tests (page 190)	
Single Leg Stand	
Sit-to-Stand	
Timed Up and Go	
Functional Reach	
Press-Up	
Squat	
1-Mile Walk	

Day 13 Another full-body session focusing on building all over strength with some of those unilateral moves we have done before. Are some of these feeling easier?

Exercises	Round 1	Round 2	Round 3
Slow Squats (with chair) (page 266)	14 reps	12 reps	10 reps
Chest Presses (page 287)	14 reps	12 reps	10 reps
Dumbbell RDLs (page 273)	10 reps each side	10 reps each side	10 reps each side
Side Lunges (page 278)	10 reps each side	8 reps each side	6 reps each side
Mountain Climbers (page 288)	10 reps each side	10 reps each side	10 reps each side
Farmer's Carry (page 289)	Walk for 30–60 secs	Walk for 30–60 secs	Walk for 30–60 secs
	REST AFTER EACH ROUND FOR 45 SECS	REST AFTER EACH ROUND FOR 45 SECS	REST AFTER EACH ROUND FOR 45 SECS

Day 14 Stretching away some possible aches from previous days. Please remember we are aiming for slow, sustainable change and progress.

Exercises	Round 1	Round 2	Round 3
Cat Cows (page 256)	8 reps	8 reps	8 reps
Bird Dog (page 259)	14 reps	12 reps	10 reps
Thread the Needle (page 257)	10 reps each side	8 reps each side	6 reps each side
Hip Flexors (page 260)	4 reps each side	4 reps each side	4 reps each side
Piriformis Stretch (page 261)	Hold 45 secs each side (count in your head if no timer)	Hold 45 secs each side (count in your head if no timer)	Hold 45 secs each side (count in your head if no timer)
Child's Pose (page 262)	30 secs	30 secs	30 secs
	REST AFTER EACH ROUND FOR 45 SECS	REST AFTER EACH ROUND FOR 45 SECS	REST AFTER EACH ROUND FOR 45 SECS

Day 15 Full-body moves here, focusing on Upper and Lower with an excellent core finish. How is the body feeling after a gentler day yesterday? Did the stretch day yesterday allow you to squat heavier?

Exercises	Round 1	Round 2	Round 3
Squats (with chair) (page 266)	14 reps	12 reps	10 reps
Bent-Over Row (page 271)	14 reps	12 reps	10 reps
Bent Arm Lateral Raises (page 272)	14 reps	12 reps	10 reps
Reverse Lunges (page 275)	10 reps each side	8 reps each side	6 reps each side
Mountain Climbers (page 288)	10 reps each side	10 reps each side	10 reps each side
Farmer's Carry (page 289)	Walk for 30–60 secs	Walk for 30–60 secs	Walk for 30–60 secs
	REST AFTER EACH ROUND FOR 45 SECS	REST AFTER EACH ROUND FOR 45 SECS	REST AFTER EACH ROUND FOR 45 SECS

Day 16 Another full-body session focusing on building all-over strength.

Exercises	Round 1	Round 2	Round 3
Squats (with chair) (page 266)	14 reps	12 reps	10 reps
Press-Ups (page 269)	12 reps	10 reps	8 reps
Hip Thrusts (page 279)	14 reps	14 reps	14reps
Reverse Lunges Biceps (page 275)	8 reps each side	8 reps each side	8 reps each side
Bikes (page 284)	10 reps each side	10 reps each side	10 reps each side
Suitcase Carry (page 290)	Walk for 30–60 secs	Walk for 30–60 secs	Walk for 30–60 secs
	REST AFTER EACH ROUND FOR 45 SECS	REST AFTER EACH ROUND FOR 45 SECS	REST AFTER EACH ROUND FOR 45 SECS

Day 17 REPEAT LONGEVITY TESTS I am excited for you to monitor and see what progress you have made. You should notice some progress, and this may be in all areas or just some. Think about why some may be more positive than others?

Tests (page 190)	
Single Leg Stand	
Sit-to-Stand	
Timed Up and Go	
Functional Reach	
Press-Up	
Squat	
1-Mile Walk	

Day 18 How are you feeling after the results yesterday? I would love to see you going heavier so we can really make good gains in our last few days.

Exercises	Round 1	Round 2	Round 3
Squat Thrusters (page 268)	14 reps	12 reps	10 reps
Bent-Over Row (page 271)	10 reps	8 reps	6 reps
Dumbbell RDLs (page 273)	12 reps	10 reps	8 reps
Reverse Lunges (page 275)	10 reps each side	8 reps each side	6 reps each side
Twists (page 285)	10 reps each side	10 reps each side	10 reps each side
Suitcase Carry (page 290)	Walk for 30–60 seconds	Walk for 30–60 seconds	Walk for 30–60 seconds
	REST AFTER EACH ROUND FOR 45 SECS	REST AFTER EACH ROUND FOR 45 SECS	REST AFTER EACH ROUND FOR 45 SECS

Day 19 Your final stretch session. Have you noticed that these have become easier, and can you feel how they complement the strength sessions?

Exercises	Round 1	Round 2	Round 3
Cat Cows (page 256)	8 reps	8 reps	8 reps
Bird Dog (page 259)	14 reps	12 reps	10 reps
Thread the Needle (page 257)	10 reps each side	8 reps each side	6 reps each side
Hip Flexors (page 260)	4 reps each side	4 reps each side	4 reps each side
Piriformis Stretch (page 261)	3–6 sets of 20 steps	3–6 sets of 20 steps	3–6 sets of 20 steps
Child's Pose (page 262)	30 secs	30 secs	30 secs
	REST AFTER EACH ROUND FOR 45 SECS	REST AFTER EACH ROUND FOR 45 SECS	REST AFTER EACH ROUND FOR 45 SECS

Day 20 As we head to the end of the 21 days with this full-body session here, focusing on Upper and Lower with an excellent core finish, please take note of how your body is feeling after a gentler day yesterday? Has the rest allowed you to squat heavier or without support?

Exercises	Round 1	Round 2	Round 3
Squats (page 265)	14 reps	12 reps	10 reps
Chest Presses (page 287)	14 reps	12 reps	10 reps
Plank Taps (page 283)	14 reps	12 reps	10 reps
Side Lunges (page 278)	10 reps each side	8 reps each side	6 reps each side
Twists (page 285)	10 reps each side	10 reps each side	10 reps each side
Farmer's Carry (page 289)	Walk for 30–60 secs	Walk for 30–60 secs	Walk for 30–60 secs
	REST AFTER EACH ROUND FOR 45 SECS	REST AFTER EACH ROUND FOR 45 SECS	REST AFTER EACH ROUND FOR 45 SECS

Day 21 FINAL DAY PLUS TEST DAY

Exercises	Round 1	Round 2	Round 3
Squats (page 265)	14 reps	12 reps	10 reps
Overhead Presses (page 280)	14 reps	12 reps	10 reps
Reverse Lunges Biceps (page 276)	10 reps each side	8 reps each side	6 reps each side
Dumbbell RDLs (page 273)	14 reps	12 reps	10 reps
Twists (page 285)	10 reps each side	10 reps each side	10 reps each side
Single-Leg Thrusts (page 279)	10 reps each side	10 reps each side	10 reps each side
Farmer's Carry (page 288)	Walk for 30–60 secs	Walk for 30–60 secs	Walk for 30–60 secs
	REST AFTER EACH ROUND FOR 45 SECS	REST AFTER EACH ROUND FOR 45 SECS	REST AFTER EACH ROUND FOR 45 SECS

FINAL LONGEVITY TESTS While this may be your final test of the plan, I would love you to keep testing every month so you can stay on top of your mobility and see measurable progress.

Tests (page 190)	
Single Leg Stand	
Sit-to-Stand	
Timed Up and Go	
Functional Reach	
Press-Up	
Squat	
1-Mile Walk	

CHAPTER 31

The Exercises

The Mobility and Balance Stretches

Bent Knee Calf Stretch
This specifically targets the soleus muscle, which sits under the gastrocnemius (main calf muscle). It is often tight in midlife and older adults due to decreased movement variety or footwear choices (heels or supportive shoes that limit ankle flexion). The stretch is crucial for improving ankle mobility, which impacts squatting, walking and even balance, and it helps prevent Achilles issues and plantar fasciitis.

How to do it: Stand facing a wall, about an arm's length away. Place both hands on the wall at shoulder height. Step one foot back (like a lunge), keeping both feet pointing straight ahead. Bend the front knee while keeping the back heel on the ground. You'll feel the stretch lower in the calf, closer to the heel.

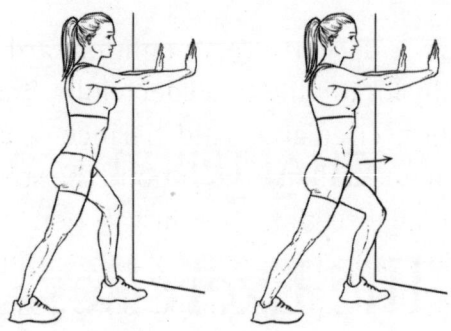

Downward Dog Knee Bend

This stretches the entire posterior chain: the calves (both soleus and gastrocnemius), hamstrings, glutes and spine. Bending one knee at a time isolates and deepens the calf stretch. Improving overall flexibility, circulation and mobility, this stretch is excellent prep for walking, running or standing workouts.

How to do it: Start in a downward dog position: hands shoulder-width apart, feet hip-width apart, hips lifted high. Your body forms an inverted V-shape with heels reaching towards the ground (they don't have to touch). Begin to bend one knee while keeping the other leg straight, pressing the straight heel towards the floor. Alternate sides slowly, like a gentle walking motion.

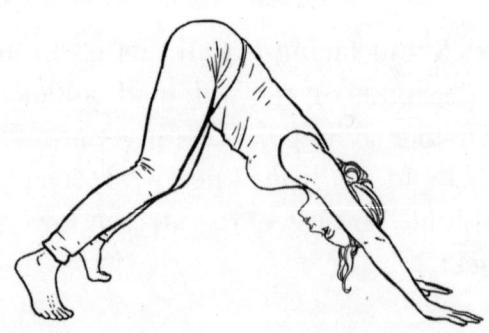

Ankle Circles

Ankle circles are a deceptively straightforward but essential exercise, especially for midlife and older adults. They help maintain joint mobility, circulation and balance – all critical for functional movement and fall prevention. The stretch improves ankle mobility in all directions (not just flexion/extension) and enhances proprioception (awareness of joint positioning) – vital for balance. It also encourages blood flow, reducing stiffness and risk of swelling, which is particularly helpful if sitting or standing for long periods. Preps the body for walking, running, squats and lunges.

How to do it:

Seated version: Sit upright on a chair, with your back supported and one leg lifted slightly off the ground. Point your toes and begin drawing large, slow circles with your foot.

Standing version: Stand on one leg (use a wall or chair for support if needed). Lift the other foot just off the ground and perform the same slow, circular movements at the ankle.

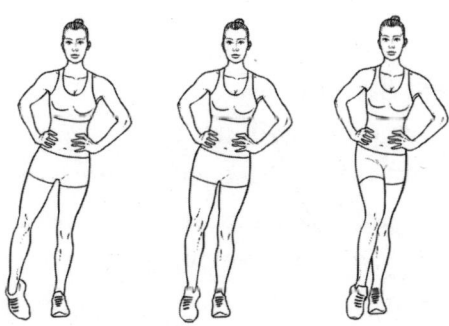

Cat Cows

The Cat Cow stretch is a simple but powerful movement that gently mobilises the spine, eases stiffness and helps connect breath with body. Perfect for mornings, warm-ups or winding down, it's a go-to exercise for improving posture and flexibility at any age.

How to do it: Start on your hands and knees, aligning your wrists underneath your shoulders. Curl your toes under. Tilt your pelvis back so that your tailbone sticks up. Your belly will drop down, but keep your abdominal muscles hugging your spine by drawing your belly button into your spine. Take your gaze gently up towards the ceiling without cranking your neck. Release the tops of your feet to the floor. Tip your pelvis forward, tucking your tailbone under. Draw your belly button towards your spine. Drop your head. Take your gaze to your belly button.

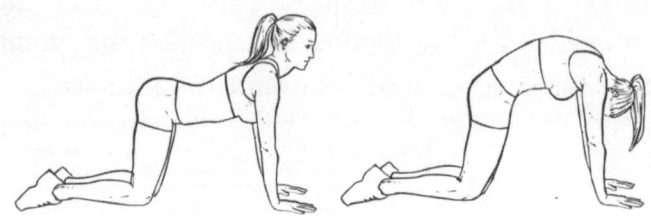

World's Greatest Stretch

This full-body, dynamic mobility drill targets the areas that often become tight as we age, including the hips, spine, hamstrings, calves and shoulders. It's excellent for joint health, circulation and preparing the body for movement. In midlife, it's especially helpful for counteracting the effects of sitting and stiffness, while improving core activation, balance and coordination. It's a simple but powerful way to support long-term mobility and keep your body moving well.

How to do it: Start in a high plank position. Step your right foot outside your right hand, landing in a deep lunge (back leg extended). Keep your left hand on the ground and rotate your right arm up towards the ceiling, opening your chest to look up at your hand. Hold for 2–3 seconds, then bring your right hand back down.

If you want, you can drop your right elbow towards your instep for a deeper hip stretch.

Shift your hips back to straighten the front leg slightly, feeling a stretch in the hamstring. Return to a high plank and repeat on the other side.

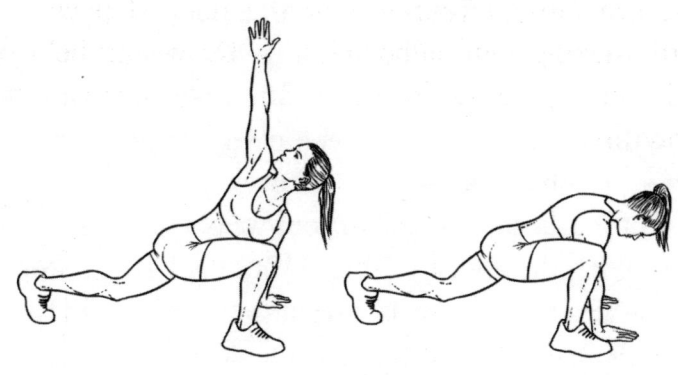

Thread the Needle

Thread the Needle is a gentle stretch that releases tightness in the shoulders, chest and upper back. It's ideal for easing tension from sitting or stress, while also encouraging spinal mobility and relaxation.

How to do it: Start on your hands and knees. Walk your right hand forward and slide the left hand between the right knee and the right hand. Twist your torso to the left and rest your head on the mat. Stay in the pose for 30 seconds, return to neutral position, reverse hands, and repeat.

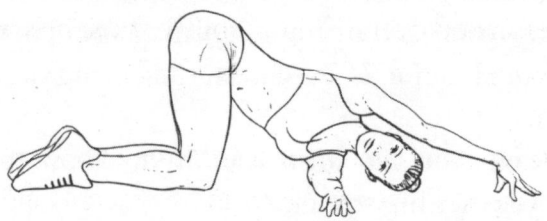

Walkouts

A walkout is a full-body plank variation that strengthens the core and shoulders while warming up the entire body. From standing, you hinge forward, walk your hands into a high plank, then return to stand. For a gentler option, drop to your knees in a plank to reduce pressure while still engaging key muscles.

How to do it: Start with your feet hip-width apart. Bending from your hips, reach for the ground and place your palms on the floor in front of your feet. Slowly shift your weight onto your hands and begin walking them forwards until your body is in a straight line from your head to your heels, bracing your core and making sure your hands are directly under your shoulders.

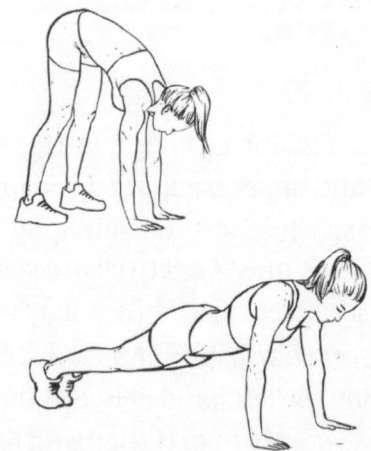

Good Morning!

This exercise is great for improving hip extension strength and building up muscle mass in your glutes and hamstrings. It can also help enhance overall hip mobility, which is essential for longevity.

How to do it: Stand with your feet hip-width apart and slightly bend your knees. Put your hands in a surrender position. Send your hips back, keep your spine neutral and squeeze your shoulder blades together. Keep sending your hips back and push your bum back as if you were shutting a cupboard with your glutes. With your chin tucked and shoulders squeezed, bend forward from the hips to around 45 degrees. Drive back up through the glutes as you come back up to standing, following the line of your legs.

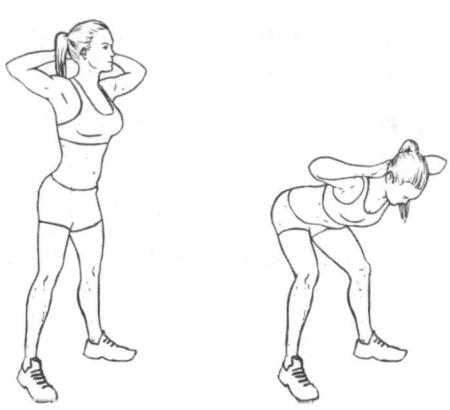

Bird Dog

The bird dog is one of the most effective core stability exercises, especially in midlife and beyond. While it may appear simple, it delivers powerful benefits. It strengthens the deep core muscles, improves posture and balance, and is gentle on the joints, making it suitable for all fitness levels. It also enhances coordination, which naturally declines with age but is essential for functional movement, daily confidence and fall prevention.

How to do it: Begin on all fours in the tabletop position. Place your knees under your hips and your hands under your shoulders. Engage your abdominal muscles to maintain a neutral spine. Draw your shoulder blades together. Raise your right arm and left leg, keeping your shoulders and hips parallel to the floor. Lengthen the back of your neck and tuck your chin into your chest to gaze down at the floor. Hold this position for a few seconds, then lower back down to the starting position. Raise your left arm and right leg, holding this position for a few seconds. Return to the starting position.

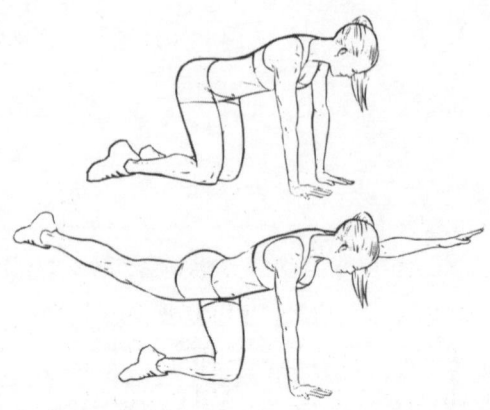

Hip Flexors

Keeping hip flexors mobile and lengthened is essential for posture, balance, back health and even pelvic alignment, which are all crucial for longevity and independence. Hip flexors are a small but mighty muscle group that tends to get tight and overworked, especially in midlife, due to more sitting, stress and sometimes less movement variety.

How to do it: Stand up straight with your arms at your sides. Place your hands on your hips or on your forward knee. Take a step forward with your right foot so you are standing in a split stance. Lower your right knee to a 90-degree angle. Extend your left leg straight back behind you. Hold the stretch for 20–30 seconds. Repeat on the other side.

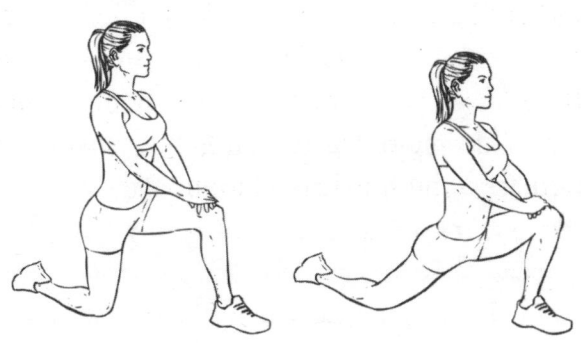

Piriformis Stretch

The piriformis stretch is a key stretch, especially for midlife women who might be experiencing tight hips, lower back discomfort or sciatic-type symptoms. The piriformis is a deep gluteal muscle that, when tight, can compress the sciatic nerve, causing pain or numbness down the leg (often called piriformis syndrome).

How to do it: Lie on your back with both knees bent and your feet flat on the floor. Put the ankle of the leg you want to stretch on your opposite thigh near your knee. Use your hand to gently push your knee (on the stretched leg) away from your body until you feel a gentle stretch around your hip.

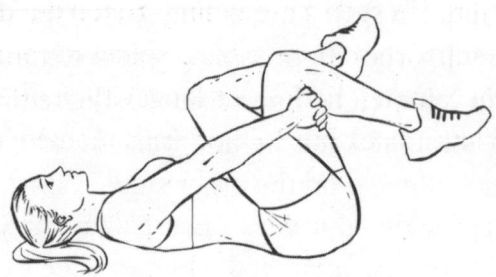

Child's Pose

This simple but deeply restorative stretch is perfect for every age and is particularly soothing for midlife women who need a moment of reconnection, release and calm. It gently stretches the lower back, hips, pelvis and inner thighs. It can help reduce tension in the spine and shoulders, especially after sitting or stress, and is great for pelvic floor awareness and gentle core release.

How to do it: Kneel on the floor with your big toes touching and knees apart (wide for hip opening, narrow for lower back focus). Sit your hips back towards your heels. Extend your arms forward, palms down, and rest your forehead on the mat. Let your chest sink towards the ground. Breathe deeply into your belly and lower back.

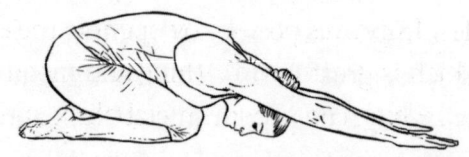

Happy Baby Pose

I love this stretch. It's such a grounding stretch but deeply powerful in how it supports hip openness, spinal decompression and nervous system calming. Perfect for longevity, it offers relief from tight hips and lower back pressure or just a moment of release.

How to do it: Lie on your back on a mat. Bring your knees in towards your chest. Open your knees wide, towards your armpits. Flex your feet and reach up to grab the outsides of your feet (or ankles/shins if you can't reach). Gently pull your feet downward while pressing your lower back into the floor. Let your hips gently open as your knees move towards the floor.

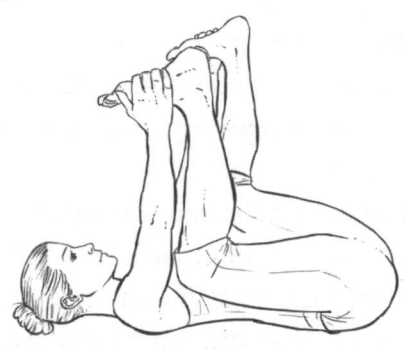

Cobra

This is a brilliant, accessible backbend that offers a gentle spinal stretch. It is especially good in midlife for those who may spend a lot of time sitting, rounding forward or dealing with tight hips and weak postural muscles. Improves posture by opening the chest, lungs and abdominals, which is great for breathing and mood. Stimulates the digestive organs, which can support metabolism and gut health.

How to do it: Lie flat on your belly, legs extended back with the tops of your feet on the floor. Place your hands under your shoulders, elbows tucked in close to your ribs. Press lightly into your hands and begin to lift your chest off the mat only as far as is comfortable. Keep your elbows bent, shoulders relaxed and down, and engage your glutes and lower abs. Gaze forward or slightly up, keeping the neck long.

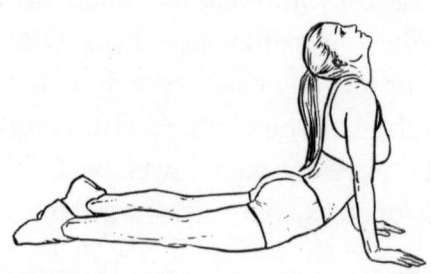

Thoracic Rotation

The thoracic rotation is a brilliant stretch for improving mobility through the middle and upper back while also releasing tension in the hips and glutes. It helps counteract the stiffness that builds up from sitting or poor posture, encouraging better spinal alignment and freer movement through the torso. Regularly practising this stretch can enhance overall posture, make daily movements feel easier, and even improve your breathing by opening up the chest and ribcage.

How to do it: Sit tall on the floor with your legs extended in front of you. Cross your left leg over your right so that your left foot is placed flat on the floor beside your right thigh. Place your left hand on the floor just behind you for support, and bring your right arm across your body, resting your right elbow on the outside of your left knee or thigh. Inhale to lengthen your spine, then exhale as you gently twist your torso towards your left side, looking over your shoulder. Hold for a few breaths, feeling the stretch through your spine and shoulders, then slowly return to centre and repeat on the other side. You can deepen the stretch by gently turning your head to look over the shoulder of your twisting side. This small adjustment enhances the rotation through your upper spine and neck, allowing for a fuller stretch across your chest, shoulders, and back. Just remember to move slowly and maintain a tall posture, avoiding any strain or forcing the movement.

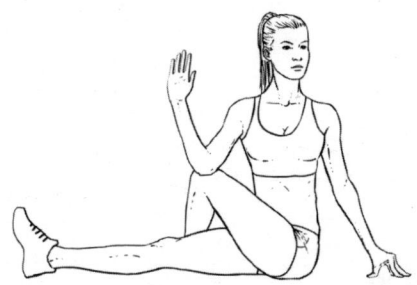

The Strength and Stability Exercises

Squats

It's hard not to notice how perfectly toddlers squat. That's because squatting is a fundamental movement pattern that requires the integration of multiple joints and muscles. As we age, we tend to forget this movement in favour of bending over.

However, incorporating squats into your exercise routine can lead to numerous benefits. Not only can squats improve your overall exercise performance, but they can also reduce your risk of injury and help you move more efficiently throughout the day.

Additionally, many of the muscles used in squats are essential for everyday activities, such as walking, climbing stairs and carrying heavy loads.

How to do it: To begin, position your feet shoulder-width apart and let your arms rest at your sides. Maintaining a strong core and upright posture with your neck in a neutral position, slowly lower your body by bending your knees and pushing your hips backwards. Pause once your thighs are parallel to the ground before standing back up and squeezing your glutes. This movement can be made more challenging by adding weight.

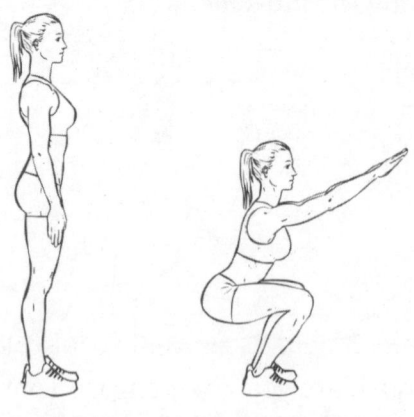

Squats (with chair)

If you need to use a chair when you begin, you can do this in two ways:

Complete beginner: You can sit in and up from a stable chair.

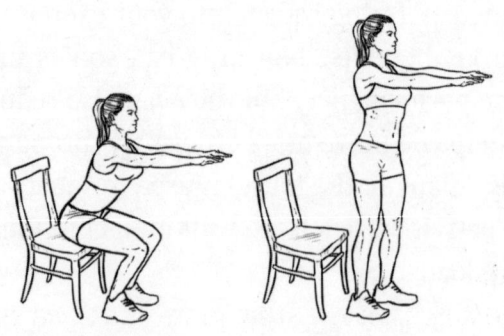

Next level: Use the chair in front to support you as you go down.

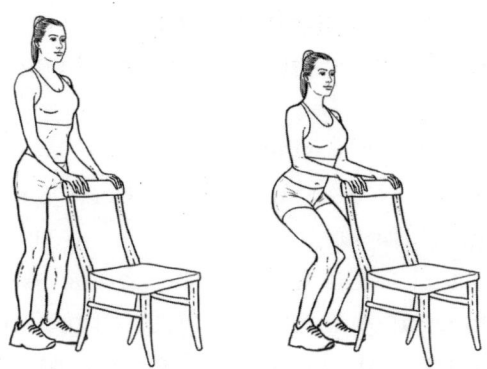

Squat Jumps

This is the same technique as above, but it explodes up from the bottom of the squat. As you land, engage your core, keep your heels on the ground, execute a squat and propel yourself back up.

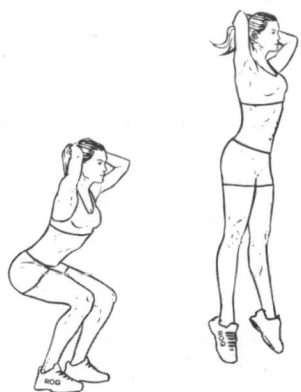

Sumo Squats

A squat is excellent for boosting glute and quad strength, but a sumo squat is even more effective for targeting the adductor, or inner thigh, muscles.

How to do it: Start in a traditional squat stance with your feet about shoulder-width apart and toes pointed forward. Take a step to the side with your right foot until your stance is about 1 metre wide, or wider than hip width.

Angle your toes out and away around 45 degrees laterally, rotating at the hip.

Move your hips back slightly and bend your knees as you lower your body into a squat position. Keep your core engaged and eyes forward throughout the movement. Lower until your thighs are parallel to the floor. If the parallel is too low or you can't maintain leg alignment, you can lower or shorten the squat.

Pause in the squat position for a few seconds. Then, engaging your glutes, press up to standing, driving up through your heels.

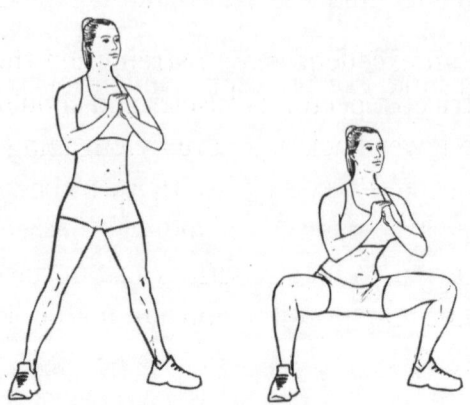

Squat Thrusters

These are a compound exercise that combine the squat with the overhead press. This is a very complete and versatile exercise that strengthens your entire body and improves your aerobic fitness, stamina and endurance.

How to do it: Stand with your feet shoulder-width apart and hold your dumbbells in front of your shoulders. Squat down until your thighs are parallel to the floor. Stand up and extend your arms over your head. Bend your arms, return to the starting position, and repeat the exercise.

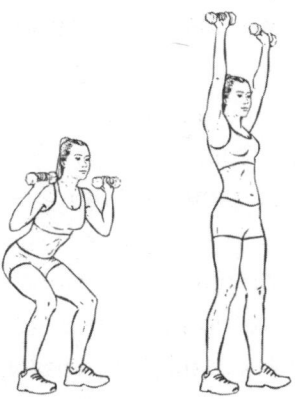

Press-Ups

Press-ups are an excellent way to strengthen the upper body, engaging the triceps, pectoral muscles and shoulders, as well as improving the lower back and core by engaging the abs. They are a convenient and easy exercise that can be done anywhere without the need for equipment, and you can begin at any level and progress as you build strength. You can start using a wall, progress to a kneeling position, and aim for a full press-up over time.

How to do it: Assume a plank position. Engage your core by contracting your abs and pulling your belly button towards the spine. Breathe in as you gradually lower yourself to the floor by bending your elbows until they form a 90-degree angle. Keep your forehead up and ensure that your chest area is positioned between your hands. As you exhale, contract your chest muscles and push yourself back up through your hands.

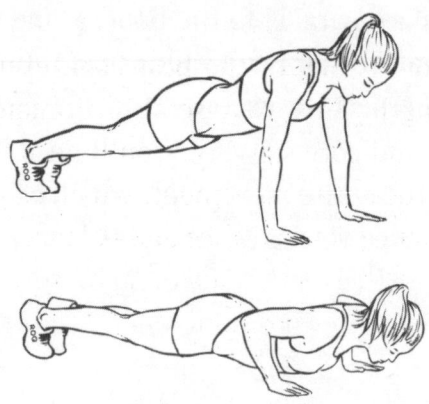

Knee Press-Ups

These are press-ups that you execute in a half position with your knees resting on the ground, rather than you whole body being used. Maintain the form as above but in a kneeling position.

How to do it: Assume an all-fours position, then engage your core by contracting your abs and pulling your belly button towards the spine. Breathe in as you gradually lower yourself to the floor by bending your elbows until they form a 90-degree angle. Keep your forehead up and ensure that your chest area is positioned between your hands. As you exhale, contract your chest muscles and push yourself back up through your hands.

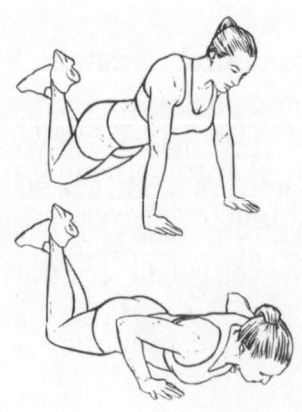

Bent-Over Row

The bent-over row is one of the best back exercises to build muscle and strength. This exercise also promotes better back posture, balance and core stability. You'll need to engage your core throughout the entire movement, which can improve your strength and enhance your posture and balance, as your core is braced throughout the movement to stabilise your upper and lower back in a bent-over position.

How to do it: Hold a dumbbell in each hand, bend your knees slightly, and hinge at the hip so your upper body is almost parallel to the floor. Keep your core tight and your back straight as you row the weights up to your chest, almost as if you are putting them into your back pocket.

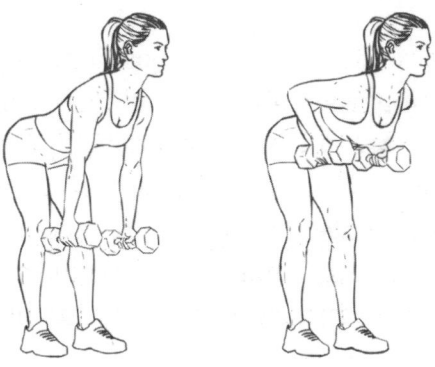

Upright Rows

An upright row is an effective exercise to build strength in the shoulders and upper back. Strengthening your posterior chain is hugely beneficial for functional everyday life.

Despite the benefits of incorporating an upright row, the exercise does have a reputation for causing injury. While this doesn't mean that you should avoid this exercise, it does mean that correct form is crucial.

How to do it: Stand with your feet shoulder-width apart, holding the dumbbells with an overhand grip down in front of you with your arms extended. Begin to lift the dumbbells, pulling through your elbows and keeping the weight close to your body as you go. Stop when your elbows are level with your shoulders and the dumbbell is at chest level. Keep your torso upright throughout the movement. Pause at the top, then return to the start.

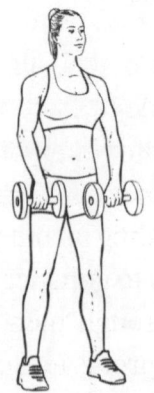
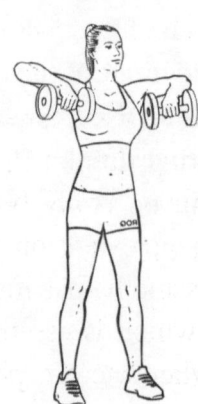

Bent Arm Lateral Raises
The bent arm lateral raise is an effective shoulder-strengthening movement. When performed regularly, it can help you develop stronger shoulders.

How to do it: Stand tall, a dumbbell in each hand. Arms are at your sides, palms facing in, elbows bent at a 90-degree angle. Position your feet roughly hip-distance apart. Check your posture – roll your shoulders back, engage your core and look straight ahead. Raise your arms to 90 degrees out to each side and pause. Breathe in as you lift. Pause and hold for a second at the top of the movement. Lower the weights, bringing your arms back to your sides. Breathe out as you lower the dumbbells.

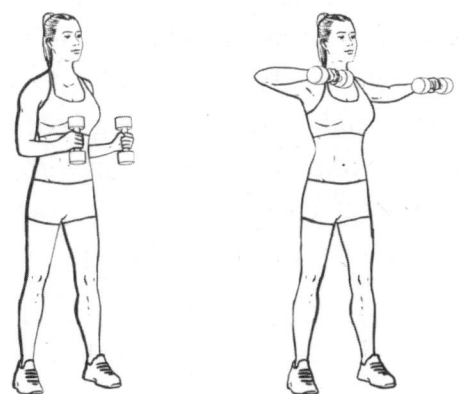

Dumbbell RDLs (Romanian Deadlifts)
Incorporating dumbbell Romanian deadlifts into your workout routine can be really beneficial. These exercises are great for improving hip extension strength and building up muscle mass in your glutes and hamstrings. They can help to enhance overall hip mobility, which is essential as we go through menopause and midlife, when we are potentially more prone to falls and hip fractures.

How to do it: Stand with your feet hip-width apart and slightly bend your knees. Take dumbbells in each hand and place them in front of your hips with your palms facing your thighs. As you send your hips back, keep your spine in a neutral position and squeeze your shoulder blades together. Keep sending your hips back and push your bum back as if you were shutting a cupboard with your glutes. With your chin tucked and shoulders squeezed, take the dumbbells following the line of your leg to halfway down on your shin. Drive up through the glutes as you come back up to standing, following the line of your legs.

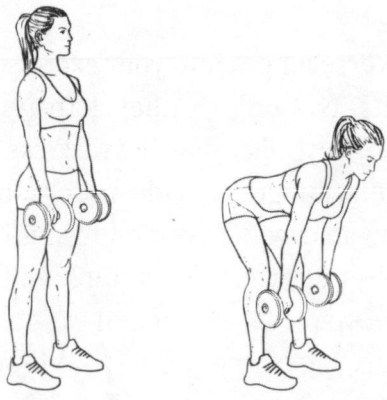

Forward Lunges

The forward lunge works your hamstrings, quadriceps, hip flexor muscles, gluteus maximus and the muscles in your inner thighs. They can help increase your stability in your core and back and are a great way to focus on balance.

How to do it: Stand tall with feet hip-width apart. Engage your core. Take a big step forward with your right leg. Lower your body until the right thigh is parallel to the floor and the right shin is vertical. Press into the right heel to drive back up to the beginning position.

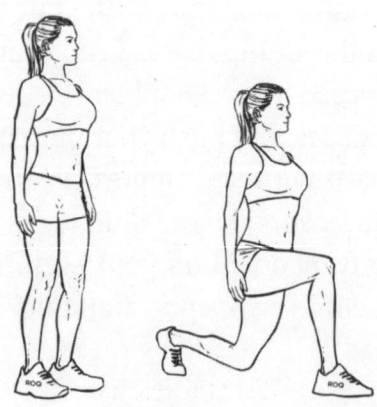

Reverse Lunges

Incorporating reverse lunges into your exercise routine can have numerous benefits. Not only do they activate your core, glutes and hamstrings, they also put less stress on your joints. Additionally, reverse lunges provide more stability in your front legs, making them an excellent option for individuals with knee concerns, difficulty balancing or less hip mobility. By switching up the direction of your movement and training your muscles to work differently, reverse lunges can help improve your balance and overall fitness.

How to do it: Stand up straight with your feet shoulder-width apart and hold a pair of dumbbells or kettlebells at your sides. Step backwards with your right leg and lunge as far as you comfortably can while dropping your hips downward. When you reach the bottom of the lunge, push back to the starting position with both legs simultaneously. Repeat the lunge with your left leg and alternate legs for the desired number of repetitions. Remember to maintain proper form and breath control throughout the exercise.

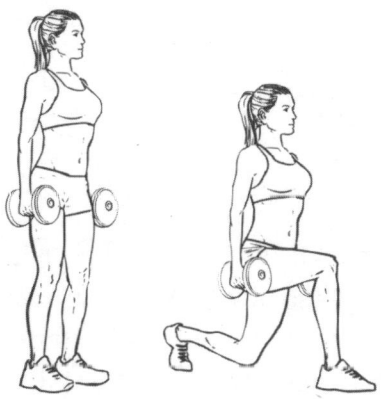

Complete beginner: Use a stable chair in front to support you as you go down and perform this exercise without weights.

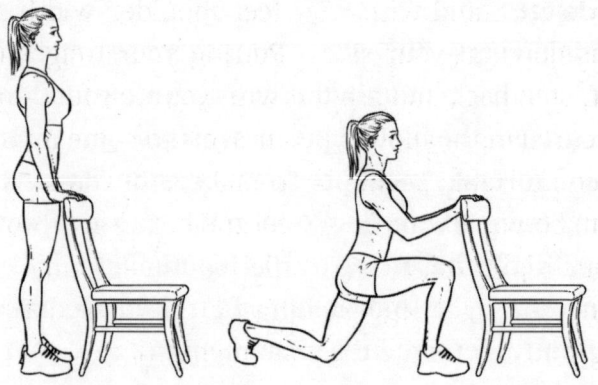

Reverse Lunges Biceps

As above but add a bicep curl for the extra challenge. As you step into the reverse lunge, lift the arms into a bicep curl.

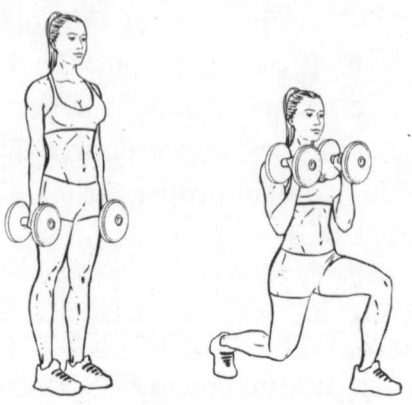

Curtsy Lunges

The curtsy lunge is great for building lower body strength and stability. The gluteus medius (GM) is an essential muscle for stability but isn't directly targeted in squats and lunges. The GM is often underactive, making strengthening exercises like the curtsy lunge even more important. Curtsy lunges also aid in strengthening the inner thigh area.

How to do it: Stand with your feet shoulder-width apart and your arms down at your sides. Putting your weight into your right foot, step back and around with your left foot – almost as if you're curtsying – allowing your arms to come up in front of you to a comfortable position. To make sure you are balanced, leave room between your front heel and bent knee. Stop lunging when your right thigh is parallel to the ground. Begin to straighten your right leg, pushing up through your heel, and returning your left foot to the starting position.

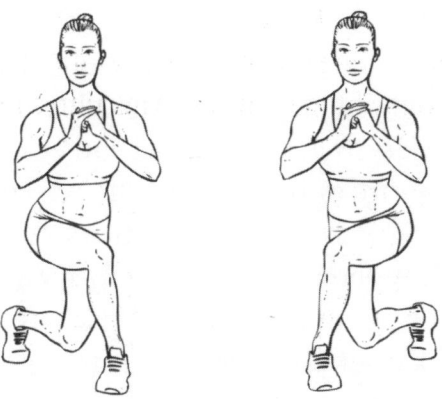

Split Squats
The split squat looks very similar to a lunge. However, during this exercise, the feet stay in one place for the most part.

How to do it: Set up in a split stance position while gripping dumbbells by your side with a neutral grip. Descend by flexing both knees simultaneously and continue until the back knee touches the ground directly beneath the hip. Drive through the front foot and extend the knee as you return to the starting position. Repeat on the other side.

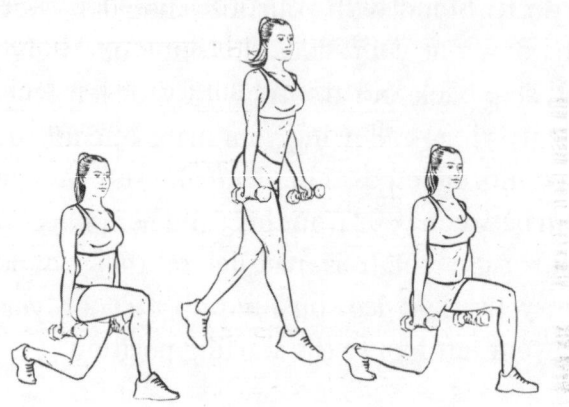

Side Lunges

One exercise that can help strengthen and improve mobility is the lateral or side-stepping lunge. Unlike traditional lunges, which move forward or backwards, this exercise involves stepping to the side. This unilateral movement is important because many of our daily activities involve only forward or backward movements. It is so important to include lateral work in your routine so we can ensure our bodies are strong and healthy enough to move in every direction, helping with balance and stability.

How to do it: Stand with your feet hip-width apart. Take a big step to the side with your left leg, then bend your left knee, push your hips back and lower until your left knee is bent 90 degrees. This should take around 2 seconds. Push back to start. Alternate sides and add weight for more strength gains.

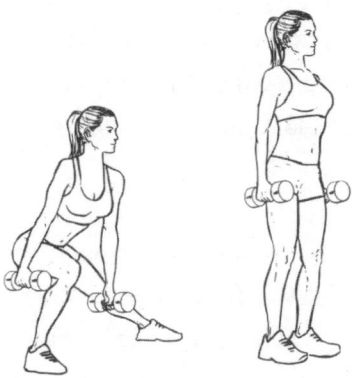

Hip Thrusts

This is a great exercise for building strength and stability. It focuses on engaging muscles in the hips, buttocks and quadriceps. If you have had a diagnosis of osteopenia or osteoporosis, this will help you target low bone density in the hips and femur bones, align your knee joints and promote better balance. It is also a fantastic way to build strong glutes and improve your fitness.

How to do it: Lie face up on the floor with knees bent, feet planted firmly on the floor and add your weight (if using) by resting across your hips. Hold the weight securely in place. Engage, brace the core and press your heels into the floor, driving your hips upwards and towards your head. Pause at the top, squeezing the glutes and lowering down, ensuring your core is engaged.

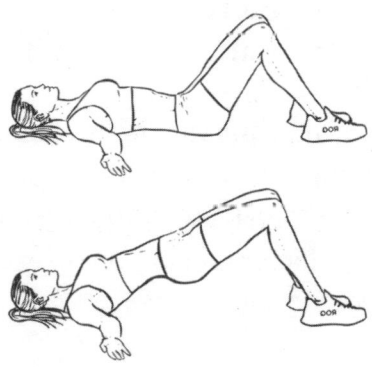

Single-Leg Thrusts

The single-leg hip thrust is a great unilateral exercise for targeting the glutes. Working each side separately isolates the glutes, which can be beneficial. This exercise has a low risk of injury and is great for all fitness levels.

How to do it: Start by lying on your back with one knee bent at about 90 degrees and the foot of the same leg flat on the floor – this will be your working leg. Lift your other leg, bending your knee until both your hip and knee form a 90-degree angle. Lay your arms out flat on the floor. Focus on using your upper back as a pivot. Contract the glute of the working leg and lift your hips until they're in line with your torso. Briefly hold this position while squeezing your glute, then return to the starting position.

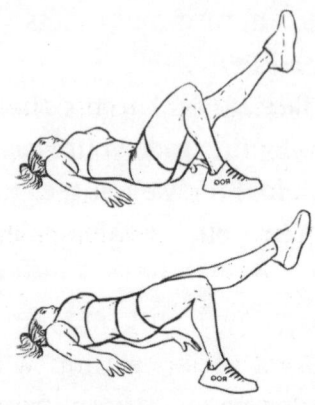

Overhead Presses

Keeping the muscles in your upper body conditioned and mobile is essential. These muscles help you perform everyday tasks, such as lifting dishes or placing items on a top shelf. To keep your upper body in shape, include the overhead press, sometimes called the shoulder press.

How to do it: Stand with your feet shoulder-width apart. Grab a pair of dumbbells and hold them at shoulder height. Ensure your spine is in a neutral position and you have a little bend in the knee. With palms facing in, drive the dumbbells overhead, then lower them slowly. Repeat this movement for your desired number of repetitions.

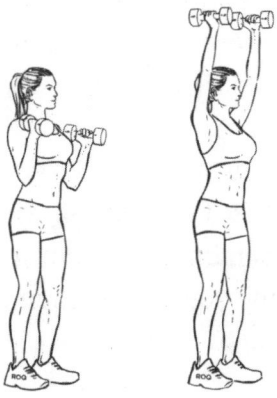

Single-Arm Overhead Presses

The single-arm shoulder press targets the shoulders, triceps and upper back, contributing to overall upper body strength. It can improve functional fitness by strengthening the muscles used in everyday activities that involve pushing and stabilising with one arm.

How to do it: Stand with your feet hip-width apart and hold your weight at a 45-degree angle away from your body. With weight in one arm, raise it up, bringing your palm forward at the top. Then, lower your arm back down to the 45-degree angle position. Use your other hand to help keep the shoulders balanced and forward.

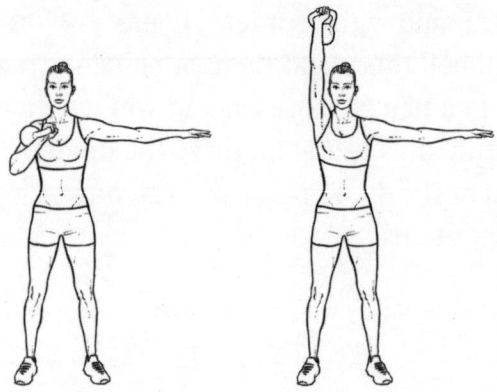

Dead Bugs

The dead bug exercise effectively strengthens and stabilises your core, spine and back muscles. This improves your posture and helps relieve and prevent lower back pain. You'll also improve balance and coordination.

How to do it: Lie on the mat with your arms extended straight over your chest so they form a perpendicular angle with your torso. Bend your hips and knees 90 degrees, lifting your feet from the ground. Your torso and thighs should form a right angle, as should your thighs and shins. This is the starting position. Engage your core, maintaining contact between your lower back and the mat. You want to ensure your spine maintains this steady and neutral position throughout the exercise. Keep your right arm and left leg exactly where they are, then slowly reach your left arm backwards, over your head and towards the floor as you simultaneously extend your right knee and hip, reaching your right heel towards the floor. Move slowly and steadily, breathing in as you perform the extensions, avoiding twisting or movement of your hips and abs. Stop the movement just before your arm and leg touch the ground.

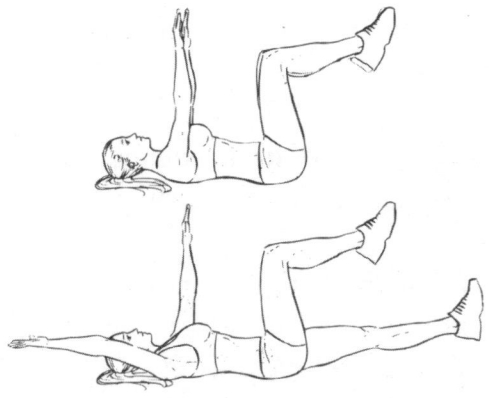

Plank Taps

Plank taps strengthen your core, glutes, arms, wrists and shoulders. This exercise helps reduce lower back pain and improves your posture and flexibility.

How to do it: Start in a plank position, with your wrists under your shoulders and your feet hip-width apart. Engage your core and touch your left shoulder with your right hand. Return to the plank and touch your right shoulder with your left hand; continue alternating sides until the set is complete.

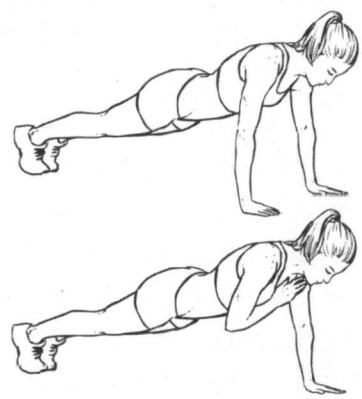

Beginner: Please do these on your knees.

Bikes

Bicycle crunches work your lower, middle and upper abs while strengthening your quads and hamstrings.

How to do it: Start by lying on the ground, with your lower back pressed flat into the floor. Place your hands lightly on the sides of your head; don't knit your fingers behind. Lift one leg just off the ground and extend it out. Lift the other leg and bend your knee towards your chest. As you do so, twist through your core, so the opposite arm comes towards the raised knee. You don't need to touch your elbow to your knee; instead, focus on moving through your core as you turn your torso. Your elbow should stay in the same position relative to your head throughout – the turn that brings it closer to the knee comes from your core.

Lower your leg and arm simultaneously while bringing up the opposite two limbs to mirror the movement. Keep on alternating.

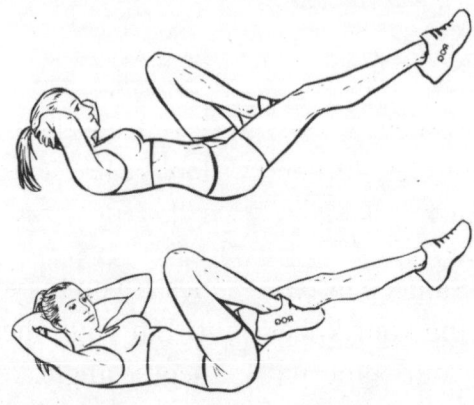

Crunch Taps

Crunch Taps are a simple but effective core exercise that targets the abdominals while adding a touch of coordination. They're great for building strength and stability through the midsection without needing equipment.

How to do it: Lie down on an exercise mat with your knees bent and arms at your sides. Bring your legs up to tabletop one leg at a time, knees bent, thighs perpendicular to the floor. Maintain a neutral spine and avoid arching or pressing your back into the floor. Begin by lowering the right foot and tapping it on the floor while the left leg remains in tabletop position. Return the right leg to tabletop and repeat with the left leg. Repeat for the desired amount of reps.

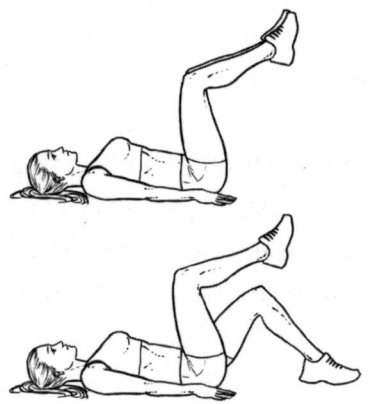

Twists

The twist is an excellent exercise for strengthening your core and shoulder muscles. Although it looks easy, it requires a lot of effort and stability.

How to do it: Sit deep into the bones as you lift your feet from the floor, keeping your knees bent. Lift your chest to the sky and straighten your spine at a 45-degree angle from the floor, creating a V shape with your torso and thighs. Reach your arms straight out in front, interlacing your fingers or clasping your hands together or holding a weight. Use your abdominals to twist to the right, then back to centre, and then to the left.

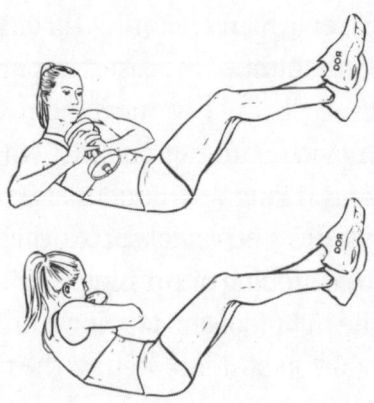

Reverse Flys

A great but challenging exercise to help you build strength in your upper back, shoulders and core.

How to do it: Stand with feet shoulder-width apart, holding dumbbells at your sides. Press the hips back in a hinge motion, bringing your chest forward and almost parallel to the floor. Let the weights hang straight down (palms facing each other) while maintaining a tight core, straight back and slight knee bend. Raise both arms out to your side on an exhale. Keep a soft bend in your elbows. Squeeze the shoulder blades together as you pull them towards the spine. Lower the weight back to the start position as you inhale. Avoid hunching your shoulders, and keep your chin tucked to maintain a neutral spine during the exercise.

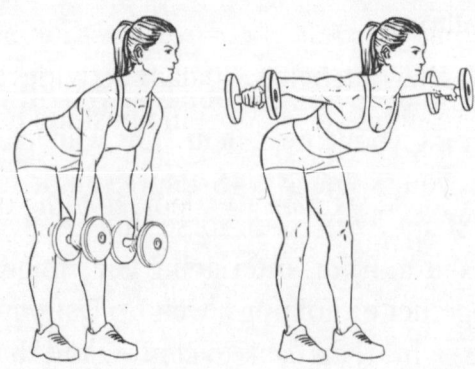

Push Presses

This is a great exercise that increases upper and lower body strength and power. By using this movement with the explosive push needed, you can help build stability and balance. It will also help build strength in your shoulders and enable you to feel more confident in lifting heavy objects overhead or having to retrieve objects from cupboards up high.

How to do it: Standing with your feet at hip width and holding dumbbells up in front of your shoulders, bend your knees slightly and lower down just a bit. Then, quickly stand up and simultaneously press the dumbbells up overhead. Keeping your glutes and core engaged is essential to stabilise your spine.

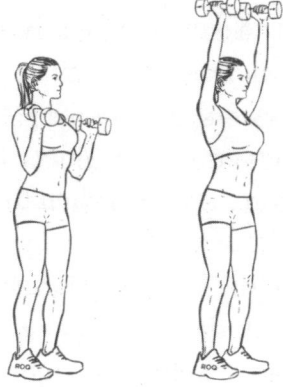

Chest Presses

These are among the best chest exercises for building upper body strength. They can help with daily activities such as carrying shopping, reaching for objects and pushing heavy doors.

How to do it: Lie face up on the floor, holding two dumbbells at chest level. Press up until your arms are fully extended. Slowly lower back to the starting position, imagining you have a sheet of glass under you as you lower your elbows steadily and in a controlled way towards the floor before powering the dumbbells back up to full extension.

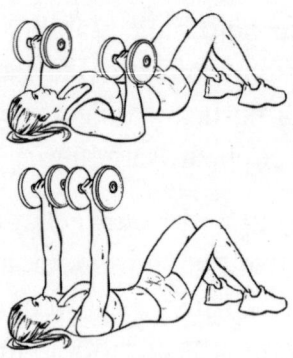

Mountain Climbers

Mountain climbers is an effective bodyweight exercise that works many muscles. Your shoulder muscles, triceps, chest muscles, serratus anterior and abdominal muscles work mainly to support your body against gravity while holding a plank position. During the exercise, your glutes, quads, hip flexors, hamstrings and calves are also recruited to move your legs.

How to do it: Start on the floor on your hands and knees. Place your hands shoulder-distance apart and align your shoulders directly over your wrists. Step your right leg back into a high plank position, aiming to keep your body straight from heel to head. Step your left leg back to meet your right leg in plank position. Keeping your neck aligned with your spine, focus on a spot on the floor just in front of your hands. Using your abdominals, bend your right knee towards your chest, then step back into the plank position. Repeat with your left leg, bringing it towards your chest and then stepping back.

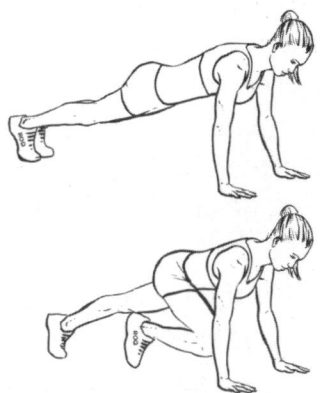

Farmer's Carry

A farmer's carry is a strength and conditioning exercise in which you hold a heavy weight in each hand and walk for a set distance or time, engaging multiple muscle groups and improving grip strength and core stability. To enhance longevity, aim to hold weights equivalent to 75% of your body weight (37.5% in each hand) for a minute.

How to do it: Grab two heavy weights (like a dumbbell or kettlebell), pick them up with a deadlift-like motion, maintain a tall posture with a braced core, and walk for a set distance or time, focusing on good form and gradual progression.

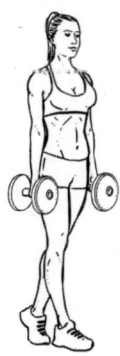

Suitcase Carry

The suitcase carry exercise offers numerous benefits for everyday life, quality of life and longevity. Strengthening the core, shoulders and grip enhances stability and balance, reducing the risk of falls and injuries in daily activities.

How to do it: Hold a weight (like a dumbbell or kettlebell) in one hand by your side, engage your core, maintain good posture and walk forwards, focusing on controlled movements and avoiding excessive arm motion.

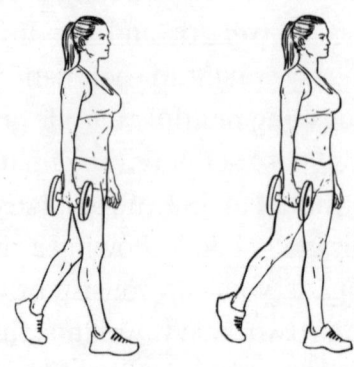

PART 5

Menus, Recipes and Meal Plans

As we move into the meal and menu plans, it's important to remember that this isn't about following a rigid set of rules. It's about showing up for yourself consistently, compassionately and with curiosity. You already understand the why behind each meal: to support your bone health, balance your hormones, energise your days and future-proof your body.

This next phase is where knowledge meets action. It's where nourishing your body becomes a lived experience: one choice, one meal, one moment at a time.

But even the most well-crafted plan is only as effective as the mindset that accompanies it. That's why this section is about more than just what to eat. It's about how you engage with your choices, and how you stay motivated without falling into the trap of all-or-nothing thinking.

We're not aiming for perfection, we're aiming for progress. The goal is to build habits that feel realistic and sustainable in your real life. That's why the recipes ahead are practical, flexible and built with busy days in mind. No endless ingredient lists, no overcomplicated prep. Just meals that nourish you, support your hormones and can be shared with family or made in batches to lighten your load.

You've already got your journalling cues. Now's the time to use them as a gentle daily check-in about your eating. You don't need to write a novel. A few short notes can make all the difference.

At the end of the day, take 2 minutes to ask yourself:

- What gave me energy today?
- What helped me feel calm or balanced?
- What made me feel a bit off, and why?

These small questions will help you make connections. Did that fibre-rich lunch keep your energy stable all afternoon? Did your sleep improve after cutting out that glass of wine? Did you feel bloated after skipping your usual protein-rich breakfast? You're not trying to get it right, you're learning your own body's rhythms.

And don't worry if you miss a day (or three). You haven't failed. You're still in motion. This is the beauty of the 21-Day Plan; it's built for real life, not ideal circumstances.

You'll notice that all the meals in this plan are meat-free, focusing on plants, legumes, whole grains, nuts, seeds and fish. This isn't just a trend; it's a deliberate choice. A mostly plant-based, pescatarian approach gives your body what it needs: fibre for gut health, antioxidants to reduce inflammation and omega-3s to protect your heart, joints and brain. If you'd like to add meat occasionally, that's your choice, but these meals give you the full support you need, just as they are. You can add your own recipes, but for the first 21 days, try to stick to this way of eating.

If you're tired, double up on dinner and save the leftovers for lunch. If the day runs away with you, breakfast-for-dinner is a perfectly balanced win.

> **What About Alcohol?**
>
> You might be wondering where alcohol fits into all of this. Blue Zones expert Dan Buettner points out that moderate alcohol, like a glass of red wine with friends, may support longevity. And yet, as we explored in the alcohol chapter (see page 133), the evidence is evolving. For many women in midlife, alcohol does more harm than good, especially when it comes to sleep, hormones and mental clarity.
>
> That's why I'm inviting you to go alcohol-free for these 21 Days. Not as a punishment, but as a reset. This is your chance to notice how you feel without it to reconnect with genuine energy, better sleep and the calm that comes from balanced blood sugar and a well-nourished nervous system.
>
> If you choose to reintroduce alcohol later, you'll be doing so from a place of awareness, not habit.

There is no right way to use this plan. Some people love prepping every Sunday and following it to the letter. Others pick and choose based on what they fancy that day. Both work. What matters most is that it supports your life.

I do, however, recommend that for success and sustainability prep is key and can help avoid mindless snacking and choices that may not optimise your health and well-being.

And remember: motivation doesn't just appear, it grows from action. Every nourishing choice reinforces your identity. You're someone who prioritises health. You're someone who honours your future self. Every time you prepare a meal from this plan, jot a note in your journal or make a mindful swap, you're sending yourself a message: I'm doing this. I'm building something better.

Let's move into the meals now, the practical fuel that will carry you through the next 21 days with strength, balance and ease.

Designed for simplicity, sustainability and satisfaction, the 21-Day Meal Plan is built from nutrient-dense, protein- and fibre-rich recipes, designed to support hormonal health, energy, muscle maintenance and gut function – all key pillars of long-term well-being.

To make your life easier, this plan balances variety with repetition, so you can batch cook – saving time and reducing food waste. You don't need a new recipe every day, you need meals you love, that nourish your body and fit your real life.

Every day includes:

- One balanced breakfast

- A simple, prep-friendly lunch

- A satisfying, wholefood dinner

Batch-cooking tips are included in each section. And feel free to swap days or repeat favourite meals.

Day	Breakfast	Lunch	Dinner
Day 1	Protein-Packed Yoghurt Bowl	Lentil & Sweet Potato Curry	Creamy Pesto Salmon with Lentils & Greens
Day 2	Chickpea & Tofu Omelette Muffins	Chickpea & Quinoa Chilli	Pesto Salmon & Roasted Veg Tray Bake
Day 3	Overnight Oats with a Protein Twist	Tofu & Veggie Stir-Fry with Brown Rice	Lentil & Sweet Potato Burrito Mix
Day 4	Make-Ahead Broccoli, Shiitake & Tofu Frittata	Hearty Vegetable Soup	Veggie Lentil Bolognese
Day 5	Spinach, Feta & Roasted Pepper Frittata	Lentil & Goat's Cheese Salad	Smoked Mackerel & Sweet Potato Fishcakes
Day 6	Protein-Packed Yoghurt Bowl	Lentil & Sweet Potato Curry	Creamy Pesto Salmon with Lentils & Greens
Day 7	Chickpea & Tofu Omelette Muffins	Chickpea & Quinoa Chilli	Pesto Salmon & Roasted Veg Tray Bake

Batch tips (Days 1–7)

- Make a double batch of the **Lentil & Sweet Potato Curry** (lunch for Day 1 and Day 6).
- Bake the **Chickpea & Tofu Omelette Muffins** and **Frittatas** ahead for grab-and-go breakfasts.
- Prep extra roasted veg with the **Pesto Salmon** to use cold for salads or wraps.

Day	Breakfast	Lunch	Dinner
Day 8	Overnight Oats with a Protein Twist	Tofu & Veggie Stir-Fry with Brown Rice	Lentil & Sweet Potato Burrito Mix
Day 9	Broccoli, Shiitake & Tofu Frittata	Hearty Vegetable Soup	Veggie Lentil Bolognese
Day 10	Spinach, Feta & Roasted Pepper Frittata	Lentil & Goat's Cheese Salad	Smoked Mackerel & Sweet Potato Fishcakes
Day 11	Protein-Packed Yoghurt Bowl	Lentil & Sweet Potato Curry	Creamy Pesto Salmon with Lentils & Greens
Day 12	Chickpea & Tofu Omelette Muffins	Chickpea & Quinoa Chilli	Pesto Salmon & Roasted Veg Tray Bake
Day 13	Overnight Oats with a Protein Twist	Tofu & Veggie Stir-Fry with Brown Rice	Lentil & Sweet Potato Burrito Mix
Day 14	Make-Ahead Broccoli, Shiitake & Tofu Frittata	Hearty Vegetable Soup	Veggie Lentil Bolognese

Batch tips (Days 8–14)

- The **Soup** and **Chilli** freeze well – make double and defrost as needed.
- Prep the **Fishcakes** ahead and store uncooked in the freezer.
- Use the same **Overnight Oats** base and vary the fruit/nut toppings.

Day	Breakfast	Lunch	Dinner
Day 15	Spinach, Feta & Roasted Pepper Frittata	Lentil & Goat's Cheese Salad	Smoked Mackerel & Sweet Potato Fishcakes
Day 16	Protein-Packed Yoghurt Bowl	Lentil & Sweet Potato Curry	Creamy Pesto Salmon with Lentils & Greens
Day 17	Chickpea & Tofu Omelette Muffins	Chickpea & Quinoa Chilli	Pesto Salmon & Roasted Veg Tray Bake
Day 18	Overnight Oats with a Protein Twist	Tofu & Veggie Stir-Fry with Brown Rice	Lentil & Sweet Potato Burrito Mix
Day 19	Make-Ahead Broccoli, Shiitake & Tofu Frittata	Hearty Vegetable Soup	Veggie Lentil Bolognese
Day 20	Spinach, Feta & Roasted Pepper Frittata	Lentil & Goat's Cheese Salad	Smoked Mackerel & Sweet Potato Fishcakes
Day 21	Protein-Packed Yoghurt Bowl	Lentil & Sweet Potato Curry	Creamy Pesto Salmon with Lentils & Greens

Batch tips (Days 15–21)

- Cook a full tray of **Roasted Veg** on Day 17 to use for multiple meals.

- Stick to familiar staples to reduce stress in the final week.

BREAKFASTS

Protein-Packed Yoghurt Bowl (Serves 1)

....

A quick, creamy bowl that packs a protein punch – perfect for busy mornings.

250g 0% fat Greek yoghurt
½ banana, mashed
1 tbsp (15g) nut butter
   (almond, peanut or your favourite)

40g blueberries (fresh or frozen)

Optional toppings
1 tsp chia seeds
1 tsp pumpkin seeds
1 tsp flaxseeds
a splash of milk (dairy or plant-based)

1. Mix the yoghurt, mashed banana, nut butter and blueberries in a bowl.
2. Sprinkle with seeds and any extras you love.

Nutritional info (approx. per serving):
- **Protein:** 32g
- **Fibre:** 6g
- **Calories:** 330 kcal
- **Fat:** 15g
- **Carbs:** 25g

Health and longevity benefits: Greek yoghurt provides high-quality protein and gut-friendly probiotics; blueberries are rich in antioxidants; nut butter offers healthy fats and vitamin E.

Chickpea & Tofu Omelette Muffins (Makes 4)

High-protein, portable egg-free muffins that make meal-prep mornings easy.

100g chickpea (gram) flour
200g silken tofu
1 tbsp (10g) ground flaxseeds
½ tsp ground turmeric
½ tsp garlic powder
½ tsp salt
50g fresh spinach, chopped
50g mushrooms, chopped
1 tbsp olive oil

1. Preheat the oven to 200°C (180°C fan/400°F). Lightly grease a muffin tin.

2. In a blender or food processor, combine the chickpea flour, tofu, flaxseeds, turmeric, garlic, salt and a splash of water. Blend into a smooth batter.
3. Stir in the spinach and mushrooms, then divide into six muffin moulds.
4. Bake for 20–25 minutes until golden and firm.

To store: Refrigerate for up to 4 days or freeze for 2 months.

On-the-go: Grab two muffins for a full serving.

Nutritional info (approx. 2 muffins per serving):
- **Protein:** 34g
- **Fibre:** 7g
- **Calories:** 290 kcal
- **Fat:** 15g
- **Carbs:** 16g

Health and longevity benefits: chickpeas and tofu provide plant protein; flaxseeds offer omega-3s; spinach and mushrooms support immune and brain health.

Overnight Oats with a Protein Twist (Serves 1)

Creamy, satisfying oats prepped the night before for a stress-free morning.

50g rolled oats
1 tbsp (10g) chia seeds
100ml milk (dairy or plant-based)

200g 0% fat Greek yoghurt
1 tsp (5g) nut butter
40g fruit (berries, banana or apple)

Optional toppings
1 tsp pumpkin seeds

extra fruit slices

1. In a jar, combine the oats and chia seeds and cover with milk.
2. Refrigerate overnight.
3. In the morning, stir in the yoghurt, nut butter and fruit, then add your chosen extra toppings.

Nutritional info (approx. per serving):
- **Protein:** 32g
- **Fibre:** 10g
- **Calories:** 380 kcal
- **Fat:** 12g
- **Carbs:** 35g

Health and longevity benefits: oats support heart health and cholesterol; chia seeds provide fibre and omega-3s; yoghurt adds gut-friendly probiotics.

Make-Ahead Broccoli, Shiitake & Tofu Frittata (Serves 4)

A savoury, protein-rich frittata that keeps well for quick weekday breakfasts.

1 tsp olive oil
2 shallots, sliced
100g Tenderstem broccoli, chopped
200g shiitake mushrooms, sliced
50g fresh spinach
2 tsp light soy sauce
400g firm tofu, cubed
12 eggs, beaten

1. Heat the oil in a large, non-stick frying pan. Sauté the shallots, broccoli and mushrooms for 3–4 minutes.
2. Add the spinach and cook until wilted, then stir in the soy sauce.

3. Scatter the tofu over the veg, pour in the eggs and cook until the edges set.
4. Transfer the pan to a hot grill and grill until golden on top, then cool slightly and slice.

To store: Refrigerate for up to 3 days.

Nutritional info (approx. per serving):
- **Protein:** 30g
- **Fibre:** 5g
- **Calories:** 290 kcal
- **Fat:** 18g
- **Carbs:** 7g

Health and longevity benefits: eggs support brain and muscle health; broccoli and mushrooms contain immune-boosting phytonutrients; tofu adds plant protein.

Spinach, Feta & Roasted Pepper Frittata (Serves 4)

A Mediterranean-style frittata that's as good cold as it is hot.

8 large eggs
500g cottage cheese
2 garlic cloves, finely chopped
30g Parmesan cheese, grated
400g fresh spinach
2 roasted red peppers, sliced
pinch of grated nutmeg
100g cherry tomatoes
150g feta cheese, crumbled

1. Preheat the oven to 190°C (170°C fan/375°F). Line a 20cm (8 inch) tin with baking parchment.
2. In a large bowl, beat the eggs with the cottage cheese, garlic, half the Parmesan, spinach, peppers, nutmeg and some black pepper.

3. Pour into the tin and top with the cherry tomatoes and the rest of the Parmesan. Bake for 25–30 minutes.
4. Add the feta, return to the oven and bake for 5–10 minutes more until golden. Cool before slicing.

To store: Refrigerate for 3–4 days.

Nutritional info (approx. per serving):
- **Protein:** 32g
- **Fibre:** 4g
- **Calories:** 330 kcal
- **Fat:** 21g
- **Carbs:** 8g

Health and longevity benefits: spinach and peppers offer antioxidants and vitamin C; eggs and cottage cheese provide protein and support muscle and cognitive function.

LUNCHES

Lentil & Sweet Potato Curry (Serves 4–6)

A warming, comforting curry packed with plant-based protein and fibre – ideal for batch cooking.

1 tbsp olive oil
1 onion, finely diced
2 garlic cloves, crushed
1 tbsp curry powder
1 tsp ground turmeric
1 tsp ground cumin
400g dried red lentils
2 medium sweet potatoes, peeled and diced
400g tin chopped tomatoes
750ml vegetable stock
200ml coconut milk
2 big handfuls of fresh spinach

1. Heat a splash of olive oil in a large saucepan and gently fry the onion and garlic until soft.
2. Stir in the spices and cook for 1 minute.
3. Add the lentils, sweet potato, chopped tomatoes, stock and coconut milk.
4. Simmer for around 25 minutes until the sweet potato is tender.
5. Stir through the spinach and cook for 5 more minutes. Season to taste.

Make-ahead tip: Keep in the fridge for 4 days or freeze in portions.

To serve: Great with brown rice or quinoa.

Nutritional info (approx. per serving):
- **Protein:** 30g
- **Fibre:** 11g
- **Calories:** 380 kcal
- **Fat:** 14g
- **Carbs:** 48g

Health and longevity benefits: lentils support blood sugar and gut health; sweet potatoes provide beta carotene; spinach offers iron and folate.

Chickpea & Quinoa Chilli (Serves 4–6)

A hearty, one-pot chilli with plenty of protein and spice. Perfect for batch prep.

1 onion, diced
2 garlic cloves, minced
1 red or yellow pepper, diced
1 tbsp olive oil or water

1 tbsp chilli powder (adjust to taste)
1 tsp ground cumin
1 tsp smoked paprika
1 tbsp tomato purée
600g tinned chickpeas, drained
600g tinned black beans, drained
400g tin chopped tomatoes
750ml vegetable stock
200g cooked quinoa

1. Sauté the onion, garlic and pepper in the oil or by adding a splash of water for 5 minutes.
2. Stir in the spices and tomato purée.
3. Add the chickpeas, beans, tomatoes, stock and quinoa.
4. Simmer for 20 minutes until thickened.

Make-ahead tip: This lasts 4–5 days in the fridge or freeze in portions.

To serve: Top with avocado and a spoon of yoghurt or serve with wholegrain bread.

Nutritional info (approx. per serving):
- **Protein:** 31g
- **Fibre:** 13g
- **Calories:** 400 kcal
- **Fat:** 10g
- **Carbs:** 50g

Health and longevity benefits: chickpeas and beans offer fibre and plant protein; quinoa contains all essential amino acids; tomatoes have lycopene, an anti-inflammatory compound.

Tofu & Veggie Stir-Fry with Brown Rice (Serves 4)

Fast, filling and full of colour – this stir-fry is perfect hot or cold.

800g firm tofu, cubed
1 tbsp soy sauce
1 tbsp cornflour
2 tbsp olive oil
200g broccoli florets
1 red pepper, sliced
1 carrot, julienned
1 tbsp sesame seeds
30g cashews
400g cooked brown rice

1. Toss the tofu with soy sauce and cornflour. Fry in a hot pan with the oil until golden, then set aside.
2. In the same pan, stir-fry the vegetables for 5 minutes until tender and crisp.
3. Return the tofu to the pan, toss with the veg, then add the sesame seeds and cashews.
4. Serve over brown rice.

Make-ahead tip: Store in containers in the fridge for up to 4 days.

To serve: Reheat or enjoy cold with a drizzle of soy or tahini dressing.

Nutritional info (approx. per serving):
- **Protein:** 30g
- **Fibre:** 8g
- **Calories:** 420 kcal
- **Fat:** 18g
- **Carbs:** 40g

Health and longevity benefits: tofu and brown rice provide complete proteins; broccoli and carrots support detoxification; cashews add healthy fats and minerals.

Hearty Vegetable Soup (Serves 4)

A comforting, thermos-friendly soup loaded with fibre and flavour.

1 onion, sliced	750ml vegetable stock
2 garlic cloves, sliced	1 tsp dried mixed herbs
2 celery sticks, thinly sliced	125g spring greens, shredded
2 carrots or yellow peppers, chopped	800g tinned butter beans, drained
1 tbsp olive oil	150g dried red lentils
400g tin chopped tomatoes	

1. Sauté the onion, garlic, celery and carrots/peppers in a hot pan with the oil for 10 minutes.
2. Add the tomatoes, lentils, stock and herbs. Simmer for 20 minutes.
3. Add the spring greens and butter beans. Cook for another 4 minutes.
4. Season with salt and pepper and serve hot.

Make-ahead tip: Keeps for 4 days in the fridge or freeze in portions.

Nutritional info (approx. per serving):
- **Protein:** 30g
- **Fibre:** 9g
- **Calories:** 260 kcal
- **Fat:** 6g
- **Carbs:** 30g

Health and longevity benefits: butter beans offer plant protein; greens and tomatoes are high in antioxidants; carrots support eye health.

Lentil & Goat's Cheese Salad (Serves 2)

A light but satisfying salad full of earthy lentils and tangy goat's cheese.

500g green lentils (e.g. Puy)
1 garlic clove, crushed
juice of ½ lemon
1 tbsp hemp seeds

2 tbsp extra virgin olive oil
20g fresh basil, torn
120g goat's cheese, crumbled
½ tbsp pumpkin seeds

1. Simmer the lentils with the garlic in a small saucepan with plenty of water for 20 minutes until tender.
2. Drain, then mix in a serving bowl with the lemon juice, olive oil and most of the basil.
3. Top with the crumbled goat's cheese, seeds and remaining basil.

Make-ahead tip: Best served at room temperature. Can be made a day ahead.

Nutritional info (approx. per serving):
- **Protein:** 30g
- **Fibre:** 8g
- **Calories:** 360 kcal
- **Fat:** 18g
- **Carbs:** 25g

Health and longevity benefits: lentils promote satiety and blood sugar balance; goat's cheese is a digestible protein source; olive oil is heart-protective.

DINNERS

Creamy Pesto Salmon with Lentils & Greens (Serves 4)

A vibrant, protein-rich dish with omega-3s, hearty lentils and creamy pesto for comfort and flavour.

4 salmon fillets
1 tbsp olive oil
1 small onion, finely chopped
2 garlic cloves, minced
1 tsp dried thyme
250g cooked green lentils (Puy or ready-to-eat)
200g spinach or kale, chopped
2 tbsp green pesto
2 tbsp crème fraîche (optional)
juice of ½ lemon

1. Preheat the oven to 200°C (180°C fan/400°F). Season the salmon with salt and black pepper and bake for 15 minutes.
2. In a pan, heat the oil and sauté the onion and garlic for 5 minutes.
3. Add the thyme, lentils and spinach or kale. Cook until wilted.
4. Stir in the pesto, crème fraîche (if using) and lemon juice. Season to taste with salt and pepper.
5. Serve the salmon on a bed of the creamy lentils.

Nutritional info (approx. per serving):
- **Protein:** 38g
- **Fibre:** 8g
- **Calories:** 470 kcal
- **Fat:** 25g
- **Carbs:** 12g

Health and longevity benefits: salmon is rich in omega-3s and vitamin D; lentils support gut and heart health; leafy greens provide essential micronutrients.

Pesto Salmon & Roasted Veg Tray Bake (Serves 4)

A fuss-free tray bake with roasted vegetables and pesto-topped salmon or tofu – satisfying and colourful.

1 courgette, sliced
1 red pepper, sliced
1 red onion, quartered
200g cherry tomatoes
1 tbsp olive oil
4 salmon fillets
4 tbsp green pesto

1. Preheat the oven to 200°C (180°C fan/400°F).
2. Toss the vegetables with the olive oil and roast for 20 minutes.
3. Add the salmon fillets, top each with 1 tablespoon of the pesto and roast for another 15 minutes.

To store: Keeps in the fridge for 2–3 days.

To serve: Pair with quinoa, couscous or new potatoes.

Nutritional info (approx. per serving):
- **Protein:** 35g
- **Fibre:** 7g
- **Calories:** 460 kcal
- **Fat:** 28g
- **Carbs:** 15g

Health and longevity benefits: salmon supports brain and heart health; tomatoes offer antioxidants; courgette provides vitamin C and potassium.

Lentil & Sweet Potato Burrito Mix (Serves 4)

A warming, family-style mix for wraps or bowls, rich in plant-based protein and fibre.

1 large sweet potato, cubed	1 tsp chilli powder
2 tbsp olive oil	400g tin green or brown lentils, drained
1 red onion, diced	
1 red pepper, chopped	400g tin black beans, drained
1 tsp ground cumin	
1 tsp paprika	

1. Preheat the oven to 200°C (180°C fan/400°F) and roast the sweet potato with 1 tablespoon of the olive oil for 20 minutes.
2. Add another splash of olive oil to a frying pan and sauté the onion, pepper and spices until softened.
3. Stir in the lentils, beans and roasted sweet potato and cook till warmed through.

To serve: Wrap in wholemeal tortillas or serve over rice with avocado and salsa.

Make-ahead tip: Freeze in batches for future wraps.

Nutritional info (approx. per serving):
- **Protein:** 25g
- **Fibre:** 12g
- **Calories:** 410 kcal
- **Fat:** 10g
- **Carbs:** 50g

Health and longevity benefits: sweet potatoes and peppers provide vitamin A and antioxidants; beans and lentils aid digestion and stable energy.

Veggie Lentil Bolognese (Serves 4)

A comforting, high-fibre pasta sauce that's perfect for batch cooking and freezing.

1 tbsp olive oil
1 onion, diced
2 garlic cloves, minced
2 carrots, grated
2 celery sticks, chopped
1 tbsp tomato purée
400g tin chopped tomatoes
150g dried red lentils
500ml vegetable stock
dried thyme and oregano, to taste

1. Add a splash of olive oil and sauté the onion, garlic, carrot and celery until soft.
2. Stir in the tomato purée, tomatoes, lentils, stock and dried herbs.
3. Simmer for 25–30 minutes until the lentils are tender.

To serve: Great with wholewheat spaghetti or courgetti.

Batch tip: Freeze in portions for midweek meals.

Nutritional info (approx. per serving):
- **Protein:** 22g
- **Fibre:** 10g
- **Calories:** 390 kcal
- **Fat:** 8g
- **Carbs:** 42g

Health and longevity benefits: lentils support gut and heart health; carrots and tomatoes reduce inflammation; celery aids hydration and digestion.

Smoked Mackerel & Sweet Potato Fishcakes (Makes 8 – Serves 4)

Smoky, savoury fishcakes with a naturally sweet base – great with salad or peas.

500g sweet potatoes, peeled
1 tbsp olive oil, plus more for frying
2 smoked mackerel fillets (approx. 200g), flaked
1 egg
1 tsp Dijon mustard
handful of chopped parsley
wholemeal flour or breadcrumbs, for coating

1. Chop the sweet potatoes into similar-sized pieces and boil until soft.
2. Mash the sweet potatoes with a splash of olive oil and a pinch of salt to taste and allow to cool (you could make them the day before).
3. Mix the mackerel, mash, egg, mustard and parsley in a bowl.
4. Shape into eight patties and coat in the flour or breadcrumbs.
5. Chill for 20 minutes, then pan-fry in the oil until golden.

To store: Store cooked or uncooked in the fridge or freezer.

To serve: Enjoy with peas, green salad or yoghurt dip.

Nutritional info (approx. per serving – 2 fishcakes):
- **Protein:** 30g
- **Fibre:** 5g
- **Calories:** 400 kcal
- **Fat:** 22g
- **Carbs:** 28g

Health and longevity benefits: mackerel is high in omega-3 fatty acids; sweet potatoes provide slow-release carbs; mustard may support digestion.

Snacks

If you get hungry in the afternoon, this might be because you aren't eating enough protein earlier in the day. When we think about living well and nourishing our body, we must fuel it with beneficial foods. So, I would like to encourage you to stay away from sugary, processed snacks and start getting into the habit of making good choices daily.

Protein Balls

handful of almonds
2 tbsp peanut butter
1 tbsp cacao nibs

6–7 Medjool dates
1 tbsp coconut oil

1. Mix together all the ingredients in a blender, roll into balls and refrigerate (keep refrigerated for a slightly chewy texture).

Apple & Nut Butter

1 apple
1 tbsp nut butter

1. Spread the nut butter onto slices of apple.

Edamame Beans

These are a great snack and can be bought frozen in bags. Once defrosted, warm them up and lightly sprinkle with sea salt.

Roasted Chickpeas

400g tin chickpeas, drained and rinsed
drizzle of extra virgin olive oil
sea salt
Optional: paprika, curry powder or other spices

1. Preheat the oven to 220°C (200°C fan/425°F) and line a large baking tray with baking parchment.
2. Spread the chickpeas on a kitchen towel and pat them dry – remove any loose skins.
3. Transfer the dried chickpeas to the baking tray and toss them with a drizzle of olive oil and generous pinches of salt.
4. Roast the chickpeas for 20–30 minutes, or until golden brown and crisp.
5. Remove from the oven and, while the chickpeas are still warm, toss with pinches of your favourite spices.
6. Store the roasted chickpeas in a loosely covered container at room temperature.

To store: Best eaten within 2 days.

Cupboard and Fridge Essentials

Oils and condiments
Dijon mustard
Extra virgin olive oil
Green pesto
Light soy sauce
Olive oil
Tomato puree

Dried herbs and spices
Black pepper
Chilli powder
Cumin
Curry powder
Garlic powder
Mixed herbs
Nutmeg
Oregano
Paprika
Salt
Smoked paprika
Thyme
Tumeric

Fruit and vegetables
Garlic bulbs
Lemons
Onions

Cupboard
Brown rice
Chickpea (gram) flour
Cornflour
Green lentils
Quinoa
Red lentils
Roasted red peppers
Rolled oats
Tinned black beans
Tinned butter beans
Tinned chickpeas
Wholemeal flour or breadcrumbs

Fridge
0% fat Greek yoghurt
Eggs
Milk (dairy or plant-based)

Miscellaneous
Cashews
Chia seeds
Flaxseeds
Ground flaxseeds
Nut butter
Pumpkin seeds
Sesame seeds
Vegetable stock cubes
Hemp Seeds

Shopping List for Days 1–7

Fruit and vegetables
1 banana
80g blueberries (fresh or frozen)
200g broccoli florets
5 carrots
4 celery sticks
300g cherry tomatoes
1 courgette
20g fresh basil
15g fresh parsley
900g fresh spinach
40g fruit (berries, banana or apple)
250g mushrooms
2 red onions
5 red or yellow peppers
2 shallots
125g spring greens
1kg sweet potatoes
100g Tenderstem broccoli

Fridge
500g cottage cheese
2 tbsp crème fraiche
150g feta cheese
120g goat's cheese
30g Parmesan cheese

Proteins
8 salmon fillets
2 smoked mackerel fillets
200g silken tofu
1200g firm tofu

Shopping List for Days 8–14

Fruit and vegetables
1 banana
40g blueberries (fresh or frozen)
200g broccoli florets
5 carrots
4 celery sticks
300g cherry tomatoes
1 courgette
2 shallots
125g spring greens
1kg sweet potatoes
100g Tenderstem broccoli

Fridge
500g cottage cheese
2 tbsp crème fraiche

20g fresh basil
15g fresh parsley
900g fresh spinach
80g fruit (berries, banana or apple)
250g mushrooms
2 red onions
5 red or yellow peppers

150g feta cheese
120g goat's cheese
30g Parmesan cheese

Proteins
8 salmon fillets
2 smoked mackerel fillets
200g silken tofu
700g firm tofu

Shopping List for Days 15–21

Fruit and vegetables
1 banana
80g blueberries (fresh or frozen)
200g broccoli florets
5 carrots
4 celery sticks
300g cherry tomatoes
1 courgette
40g fresh basil
15g fresh parsley
900g fresh spinach
80g fruit (berries, banana or apple)
250g mushrooms
2 red onions
5 red or yellow peppers

2 shallots
125g spring greens
1kg sweet potatoes
100g Tenderstem broccoli

Fridge
500g cottage cheese
2 tbsp crème fraiche
150g feta cheese
240g goat's cheese
30g Parmesan cheese

Proteins
8 salmon fillets
2 smoked mackerel fillets
200g silken tofu
700g firm tofu

WHAT DOES THE FUTURE HOLD?

Congratulations.

You've done something extraordinary. You've committed to 21 days of nourishing your body, building strength and reconnecting with your mind. But this isn't the end. It's the beginning of a lifestyle, a new way of being that is rooted in vitality, self-awareness and joy.

Over the last few weeks, you've built habits that reflect who you are at your core. Someone who shows up, even on the hard days. Someone who moves with intention, eats with purpose and creates space for rest and reflection. You've shifted from reactive to proactive, from surviving to thriving.

This wasn't a seasonal reset or a temporary fix. This was a reclamation of your time, energy and self-worth. You didn't just learn how to eat better or move more. You learned how to listen to yourself and honour what your body needs. That is powerful.

Now, let's talk about where you go from here.

Before you look ahead, take a moment to look back. Ask yourself what surprised you. What did you enjoy the most? When did you feel your strongest, calmest, most energised self? What will you take with you into the next season of life?

Maybe it was the feeling of strength after lifting weights. The clarity that came after consistent sleep. The pride of fuelling your body with foods that make you feel good. Maybe it was the joy of dancing in your kitchen or the calm of a mindful walk.

These moments matter. They are your proof. Let them be your motivation.

You now have a toolkit to support your well-being, not just in a 21-day window, but in the months and years to come. You've learned how to fuel your body with colourful, protein-rich, whole foods. You've let go of rigid dieting and embraced balance. You've built physical strength to support ageing with confidence. You've prioritised sleep, mental resilience and emotional regulation.

If you enjoyed the programme, you could do it again. And you can, if you haven't already, buy *Owning Your Menopause: Fitter, Calmer, Stronger in 30 Days* and join that programme.

Using SMART

Now that you're looking to the future, shape your intentions into SMART goals, so that you stop relying on willpower and start using the structure you have built. This clarity helps you stay on track, continuing to build confidence, especially in midlife when your time, energy and body may feel pulled in many directions.

Setting SMART goals also encourages consistency over perfection, which is exactly what the 21-Day Plan is built on.

So, whatever you have learned and want to take on from this programme, whether it's improving sleep, increasing protein at breakfast or walking daily for energy and mood, make your goal SMART. Make it count. You're not just ticking a box; you're building a stronger, future-proofed foundation.

- Specific
- Measurable
- Achievable
- Relevant
- Time-bound

These aren't vague intentions like eat better or get fitter. They are clear, intentional commitments to the life you want to lead. Rather than relying on short-term motivation, you'll be guided by structure and clarity. This approach turns good intentions into actions and actions into sustainable habits.

Here's how to apply that structure to the pillars you've already begun strengthening.

From Habit to Lifestyle: Your SMART Goal Framework

Use this table to help shape your own realistic goals based on what you've already built. Personalise them to suit your routine and needs.

Pillar	Focus	SMART Goal Example
Movement	Build strength, improve mobility and consistency	I will strength train for 30 minutes three times a week Monday Wednesday Friday for the next 6 weeks
Nutrition	Increase fibre and protein for energy and balance	I will include 30 grams of fibre daily by adding vegetables, pulses or oats to two meals a day
Mental Well-being	Boost emotional regulation and rest	I will do a 10-minute wind-down routine including deep breathing and no screens before bed five nights a week
Journalling	Support awareness and integration across all pillars	I will try to journal for 5 minutes each evening to reflect on movement, food choices and mood

Your journal isn't just a place to track habits. It is a space to process your growth. Keep documenting what's working, what's shifting and what feels off. Use it to reconnect with your why and to spot patterns that support or sabotage your wellbeing. You don't need to write every day, but staying in the habit of checking in with yourself builds powerful awareness. Let journalling evolve into a long-term self-coaching tool that helps you adapt, stay focused and thrive.

You've discovered the power of movement feels good. Keep leaning into that. It doesn't need to be long, intense or complicated. Go heavier. Try something new. Walk more often. Dance. Stretch longer. The more you associate movement with feeling empowered, the more naturally it will fit into your life. Let it be an expression of gratitude not obligation. If you haven't already, you could buy my first book *Owning Your Menopause: Fitter, Calmer, Stronger in 30 Days* and expand deeper into the strength side of your journey.

A little structure can prevent a lot of stress. Spend 10 minutes each Sunday planning your workouts, meals and moments of rest. Diarise it but anticipate obstacles. You don't need rigid routines; just a rhythm that helps you stay grounded when life feels chaotic.

When things don't go to plan don't scrap the week. Adjust. Re-centre. Move forward.

When the novelty wears off, your Why becomes your compass. What made you pick up this book in the first place? What kind of life are you choosing now? Whether it's being active for your kids, preventing illness, reclaiming confidence or simply wanting to feel strong and capable, you have a reason. Keep it close. Write it down. Say it out loud. Let it guide your choices even on the toughest days. It's not motivation you need, it's meaning.

Every choice you've made is about more than just you. Your commitment influences your partner, your children, your friends, even your parents. You're breaking cycles, rewriting narratives and proving that it's never too late to prioritise well-being.

Conclusion: Creating Your Own Blue Zone

At the start of this book, I spoke about the Blue Zones. What makes them unique isn't a single secret or magic solution, but the way their daily habits, environment and connections naturally support longevity.

Over the past 21 days, you've seen how those same principles can be woven into your own life. Through movement, nourishment and mindful well-being, you've laid the foundations of your very own Blue Zone right at home.

But this plan was never meant to be the finish line. These 21 days are the starting point, a chance to experiment, reset and begin shaping habits that will carry you forward. Longevity isn't created in 3 weeks; it's cultivated through the small, intentional choices you repeat over months and years. Each time you cook a nourishing meal, strengthen your body, prioritise recovery or connect with someone you care about, you are reinforcing the lifestyle that supports health and vitality.

You don't need to live in Sardinia, Okinawa or Nicoya to thrive. You already have the power to create your own Blue Zone, wherever you are. I hope that this journey has shown you that longevity is not something distant or reserved for others; it is available to you, here and now.

As you move forward, keep treating your home, your habits and your relationships as the foundation for a longer, stronger, more fulfilling life. And remember, when you commit to living this way, you're not just transforming your own health, you're creating ripples of change that touch your family, your friends and your wider community.

This is the proper longevity solution: a lifelong commitment to building a life that doesn't just last longer, but feels richer, calmer and more connected one day at a time.

Write to Your Future Self

As a final act of reflection, write a letter to the version of you 6 months from now. Remind her how far you've come. Tell her what you hope she's still doing. Reconnect her to your Why. Let her know that she's capable, worthy and powerful.

Seal it. Keep it safe. Return to it when you need to remember who you are.

There is no finish line here. There is no after. There is only now and the choices you make each day to move with strength, eat with love and live with intention.

You've stepped off the yo-yo and onto a steady path. You've proven that change is possible at any age, at any stage.

So, keep going. Keep choosing you. One decision, one habit, one empowered day at a time.

ENDNOTES

1. www.alzheimers.org.uk/blog/why-dementia-different-women
2. https://pmc.ncbi.nlm.nih.gov/articles/PMC4822264/
3. www.ons.gov.uk/peoplepopulationandcommunity/healthandsocialcare/healthandlifeexpectancies/bulletins/healthstatelifeexpectanciesuk/2017to2019
4. www.ons.gov.uk/peoplepopulationandcommunity/healthandsocialcare/healthinequalities/bulletins/healthstatelifeexpectanciesbyindexofmultipledeprivationengland/2018to2020
5. www.ons.gov.uk/peoplepopulationandcommunity/healthandsocialcare/healthandlifeexpectancies/bulletins/ukhealthindicators/2019to2020
6. www.ons.gov.uk/peoplepopulationandcommunity/birthsdeathsandmarriages/deaths/bulletins/dementiaandalzheimersdiseasedeathsincludingcomorbiditiesenglandandwales/2019registrations
7. https://pmc.ncbi.nlm.nih.gov/articles/PMC11954733/
8. https://orwh.od.nih.gov/toolkit/recruitment/history
9. https://www.health.harvard.edu/blog/understanding-heart-attack-gender-gap-201604159495
10. https://pmc.ncbi.nlm.nih.gov/articles/PMC9043984/
11. https://www.mymenopausecentre.com/lifestyle-changes/lifestyle-adjustments-for-menopause/optimising-menopause-wellness-fine-tuning-hrt-dosage-for-lifestyle-balance/
12. https://pmc.ncbi.nlm.nih.gov/articles/PMC12256231/
13. https://www.kearney.com/about/strategic-partnerships/world-economic-forum/article/womens-health-the-research-gap-that-costs-lives

14 https://www.hriuk.org/health/learn/cardiovascular-disease/women-and-heart-disease
15 https://www.nhs.uk/tests-and-treatments/cervical-screening/when-youll-be-invited/
16 https://www.nhs.uk/tests-and-treatments/breast-screening-mammogram/when-youll-be-invited-and-who-should-go/
17 https://www.endocrine.org/patient-engagement/endocrine-library/menopause-and-bone-los
18 https://www.nhs.uk/conditions/high-blood-pressure/
19 https://cks.nice.org.uk/topics/melanoma
20 https://my.clevelandclinic.org/health/diseases/21608-perimenopause
21 https://pmc.ncbi.nlm.nih.gov/articles/PMC11785355/
22 https://thebms.org.uk/wp-content/uploads/2025/09/02-BMS-ConsensusStatement-BMS-WHC-2020-Recommendations-on-HRT-in-menopausal-women-SEPT2025-A.pdf
23 https://www.nia.nih.gov/health/brain-health/cognitive-health-and-older-adults
24 www.ncbi.nlm.nih.gov/books/NBK64800/
25 https://www.health.harvard.edu/staying-healthy/dont-let-muscle-mass-go-to-waste
26 https://womeninsport.org/wp-content/uploads/2021/05/Research-Report-Inspiring-Women-to-be-Active-During-Midlife-and-Menopause.pdf
27 https://pmc.ncbi.nlm.nih.gov/articles/PMC6557987/
28 https://pmc.ncbi.nlm.nih.gov/articles/PMC9235827/
29 https://www.businessinsider.com/guides/health/fitness/weight-lifting-myths-for-women
30 https://www.leedsbeckett.ac.uk/blogs/carnegie-xchange/2024/12/exercise-snacking/
31 https://pubmed.ncbi.nlm.nih.gov/38190022/
32 https://pmc.ncbi.nlm.nih.gov/articles/PMC9934205/
33 https://pmc.ncbi.nlm.nih.gov/articles/PMC10711335/
34 Ibid.
35 https://pmc.ncbi.nlm.nih.gov/articles/PMC4889622/
36 https://pmc.ncbi.nlm.nih.gov/articles/PMC4035379/
37 https://www.who.int/news-room/fact-sheets/detail/cardiovascular-diseases-(cvds)

38 https://doi.org/10.1093/eurjpc/zwad229
39 https://pmc.ncbi.nlm.nih.gov/articles/PMC12043657/
40 https://pmc.ncbi.nlm.nih.gov/articles/PMC12209867/
41 https://www.ox.ac.uk/news/2021-07-21-red-and-processed-meat-linked-increased-risk-heart-disease-oxford-study-shows
42 https://hsph.harvard.edu/news/red-meat-consumption-associated-with-increased-type-2-diabetes-risk/
43 https://www.who.int/news-room/questions-and-answers/item/cancer-carcinogenicity-of-the-consumption-of-red-meat-and-processed-meat
44 https://www.bbc.com/news/magazine-30351406
45 https://pmc.ncbi.nlm.nih.gov/articles/PMC3098911/
46 https://pubmed.ncbi.nlm.nih.gov/33803407/
47 https://www.bbc.co.uk/food/articles/improving_gut_health
48 https://www.frontiersin.org/journals/nutrition/articles/10.3389/fnut.2025.1580753/full
49 https://pmc.ncbi.nlm.nih.gov/articles/PMC8839325/
50 Table courtesy of Katie Skrine
51 https://bmjgroup.com/new-evidence-links-ultra-processed-foods-with-a-range-of-health-risks/
52 https://jamanetwork.com/journals/jamanetworkopen/fullarticle/2802963
53 https://pmc.ncbi.nlm.nih.gov/articles/PMC10879547/
54 https://news.harvard.edu/gazette/story/2017/04/over-nearly-80-years-harvard-study-has-been-showing-how-to-live-a-healthy-and-happy-life/
55 https://pmc.ncbi.nlm.nih.gov/articles/PMC11403199/
56 https://pmc.ncbi.nlm.nih.gov/articles/PMC6853739/
57 https://www.bristol.ac.uk/news/2022/june/tne-second-one-legged-stance.html
58 https://confluenthealth.com/resources/leg-strength-the-foundation-of-functional-longevity
59 https://jamanetwork.com/journals/jamanetworkopen/fullarticle/2724778
60 https://pmc.ncbi.nlm.nih.gov/articles/PMC7700832/
61 https://www.uclahealth.org/news/article/taking-walk-after-eating-can-help-with-blood-sugar-control

INDEX

abdominal fat 47, 107
Achilles tendon 221
aerobic exercise 70, 71–2, 74, 77–8
affirmation journalling 168
ageing: bone health 84–5
   brain health 88
   heart health 87–8
   hormones and 28, 31, 45–50, 83–4
   joint health 86
   metabolic health 88–9
   mitochondrial dysfunction 90
   movement and mood 89
   muscles 86–7, 89–91
   redefining 51–3
alcohol 133–6, 181, 293
almonds: protein balls 312
Alzheimer's disease 9, 18, 71, 109
anaerobic exercise 70, 72–4, 76, 77–8
ankle circles 221, 255
anti-inflammatory diet 106, 107, 111
antioxidants 101, 110
anxiety 18, 89, 135
appetite control 97

apple & nut butter 312
arthritis 18
asthma 18

back pain 188
bacteria *see* gut microbiome
balance 70, 82, 186, 231
   health assessment 190–3
   stretches 253–65
barre exercises 79
batch cooking 295–6
BDNF (brain-derived neurotrophic factor) 88
beans 103
bending 188
bent arm lateral raises 272–3
bent knee calf stretch 221, 253–4
bent-over row 271
biceps, reverse lunges 276
bikes exercise 284
bird dog 259–60
blended families 59–60
blood pressure 37, 43–4, 71, 87
blood sugar levels 71, 96, 97, 105–7, 120, 180, 230
Blue Zones 2, 19–24, 103–4, 133–4, 135, 155, 321
bolognese, veggie lentil 310–11

bones: density 28, 41–2, 84–5
  fractures 42, 84, 186
  osteopenia 27–8
  osteoporosis 9, 32, 34, 42, 45, 47, 84
bowel cancer 35–6, 40–1
brain: brain fog 34, 83, 88, 110, 111
  exercise and 71, 150
  gut-brain axis 113, 114–15
  journalling 161
  music and 173
  nutrition 109–12
  sleep 180
breakfast 235–6, 294–301
breast cancer 18, 33, 39–40
breathwork 231–2
broccoli, shiitake & tofu frittata 299–300
Buettner, Dan 19, 21, 133, 293
bullet journalling 164

caffeine 180
calcium 84, 85, 126
calf stretches 221, 253–4
California 24
cancer: bowel cancer 35–6, 40–1
  breast cancer 18, 33, 39–40
  diet and 102
  movement and 70
  skin cancer 44
carbohydrates 96–7, 100, 103, 180
cardio training 81, 90
cardiovascular disease 18, 42–3, 45, 47, 87, 102

cardiovascular system 71
caregiving 55–7, 60
cartilage 86
cat cows 222, 256
cells, intermittent fasting 121–2
cervical screening 37, 38–9
chair stand test 193–5, 208
cheese: lentil & goat's cheese salad 306
  spinach, feta & roasted pepper frittata 300–1
chest presses 287–8
chickpeas: chickpea & quinoa chilli 302–3
  chickpea & tofu omelette muffins 297–8
  roasted chickpeas 313
child-free people 59
child's pose 222, 262
children: relationship with 56–7
  single and solo parents 58
chilli, chickpea & quinoa 302–3
cholesterol 37, 43, 87
chronic illnesses 18
clinical trials 32–4
clothes 214
cobra 222, 263–4
cognitive decline 45, 88, 106, 109–12
communication 57
cooling down 210, 222–3, 234
core exercises 82
cortisol 96, 105–6, 145, 153, 171–2
Costa Rica 23
cravings 98
Crohn's disease 36

crunch taps 284–5
curry, lentil & sweet potato 301–2
curtsy lunges 276–7
cycling 78
cytokines 89, 90

daily routine 235–6
dancing 78
dates: protein balls 312
dead bugs 282–3
dementia 9, 18, 32, 34, 71, 88, 109, 110
depression 18, 89, 111
diabetes 18, 44, 45, 47, 70, 80, 88, 102, 106
digestive system *see* gut microbiome; nutrition
dinner 236, 294–6, 307–12
disease, epidemiology 17–25
DNA 10, 139
dopamine 89, 150, 171, 172
downward dog knee bend 221, 254–5
drugs, clinical trials 32
dumbbell RDLs 273–4
dumbbells 213, 219

edamame beans 313
eggs: frittatas 299–301
emotions: emotional resilience 140, 143–7
  emotional rest 176–7
  journalling 161
empty nest syndrome 57
endometriosis 33
endorphins 70–1, 89, 150, 186

energy levels 89–90, 96, 98
epidemiology 17–25
equipment 213
exercise 64, 67–91
  21-Day Plan 210, 217–23, 229–32, 237–51
  and brain health 88
  cooling down 210, 222–3, 234
  exercise snacking 79–82
  and gut health 116
  and heart health 87
  and joint health 86
  and mental health 149–52
  and mitochondria 90
  mobility and balance stretches 253–65
  and mood 89
  music and 173
  resistance training 6, 28, 67, 72–4
  warm-ups 209–10, 220–1, 234, 235

falls 70, 84–5, 86, 186, 190
farmer's carry 231, 289
fasting, intermittent 119, 121–3
fat, abdominal 47, 107
fatigue 89
fats, in diet 98, 100
fibre 99, 100, 101, 103, 114, 117
fish 102
fishcakes, smoked mackerel & sweet potato 311–12
flexibility 70, 74–5, 78–9, 82
folate 127
forward lunges 274

fractures 42, 84, 186
friends 6–7, 60, 151, 153–7
frittatas 299–301
fruit 314–16
functional fitness 183–208
functional reach test 198–200, 208

GABA 115, 145
gait 188
gender health gap 32–4
goals 318–21
Good Morning! exercise 221, 259
gratitude journalling 163
Greece 23
grip strength 231
growth hormones 86
The Guardian 33
gut microbiome 113–18
   alcohol and 135
   fibre and 101, 103
   gut-brain connection 114–15
   intermittent fasting 122
   and sleep 180–1
   ultra-processed foods and 130
gut problems 18, 36

hamstrings 221
happy baby pose 222, 263
health and habit journalling 167, 170
health assessment 183–208
healthspan 10, 27–9, 186
heart disease 17–18, 32, 37, 44, 47, 69, 106
heart health 42–3, 87

HIIT (High-Intensity Interval Training) 73, 74, 76, 90
hinge movement 188
hip flexors 260–1
hip fractures 84
hip thrusts 279
hormone replacement therapy 33, 48–9, 84
hormones: and ageing 28, 31, 45–50, 83–4
   alcohol and 134
   menopause 48–50, 83
   and mental health 143–7, 151
   nutrition and 93, 98, 103
   stress hormones 96, 105–6, 153, 171–2
hunger 120
hydration 112, 214

IBS 18
Ikaria, Greece 20, 23, 103, 133
immune system 88–9, 90, 113
incontinence 18
inflammation 71, 73, 87, 90, 91, 106, 110, 111, 120, 121
insulin 88, 91, 105
insulin resistance 47, 135
intermittent fasting 119, 121–3
iron 99
isolation 153–4
Italy 21, 22

Japan 22–3
joints: and ageing 67
   joint health 86
   mobility 75
   pain 18

INDEX 331

journalling 64–5, 141, 159–70, 181, 234
   21-Day Plan 210, 216, 225–8
joy 141

legs: squats 185, 187, 203–5, 208, 230, 265–9, 277–8
   strength 230
   stretches 221, 253–4
lentils: creamy pesto salmon with lentils & greens 307–8
   lentil & goat's cheese salad 306
   lentil & sweet potato burrito mix 309–10
   lentil & sweet potato curry 301–2
   veggie lentil bolognese 310–11
LGBTQ+ people 58–9
life expectancy 18
lifespan 9, 10, 19–25, 27–9
LII (Low-Intensity Steady State) Cardio 77
liver 103
Loma Linda, California 24, 103–4
loneliness 153–4
lunch 236, 294–6, 301–6
lunges 186, 187, 274–9

macronutrients 96–9, 100
magnesium 99, 110, 127, 180
mats 213
meat 102–4
Mediterranean diet 22
melanoma 44
memory problems 110

men: ageing 51
   clinical trials 32–4
menopause 45–50
   and bone health 42
   effects on brain 111
   gender health gap 34
   hormones 48–50, 83
mental health 6, 64, 139–82
   exercise and 70–1, 149–52
   gut-brain axis 113, 114–15
   hormones and 143–7
   journalling 159–70
   mindful eating 120–1
   music 171–4
   rest and recovery 175–8
   sleep 181
   social connections 153–7
metabolism 88–9, 121
micronutrients 99–100
migraine 18
mindful eating 119–21
minerals 110
mitochondria 81, 89–90
mobility: exercises 70, 74–5, 78–9, 82
   functional fitness 186
   health assessment 190
   stretches 253–65
   warm-ups 209–10
moles 44
mood, movement and 89
morning pages, journalling 165–6
Mosconi, Dr Lisa 88
motivation, 21-Day Plan 214
mountain climbers 288–9
movement *see* exercise

muffins, chickpea & tofu omelette 297–8
muscles: ageing 28, 67
　flexibility 74–5
　functional fitness 185–8
　imbalance 218
　muscle health 86–7
　myokines 91
　strength training 70, 72–4, 219–20
mushrooms: broccoli, shiitake & tofu frittata 299–300
music 141, 171–4
myokines 89, 91

National Geographic 21
National Institute for Health and Care Excellence (NICE) 84
National Institutes of Health (NIH) 32
neurotransmitters 115, 144, 181
neurotrophins 71
Nicoya Peninsula, Costa Rica 23, 103
nut butter, apple & 312
nutrition 6, 64, 93–137
　21-Day Plan 214–15
　alcohol 133–6
　anti-inflammatory diet 106, 107
　cupboard and fridge essentials 314
　gut microbiome 113–18
　intermittent fasting 119, 121–3
　menus, recipes and meal plans 291–316
　mindful eating 119–21
　shopping lists 315–16
　supplements 125–7
　to slow cognitive decline 109–12
　ultra-processed foods 129–32

oats: overnight oats with a protein twist 298–9
oestrogen: and bone health 42
　and brain health 88
　and cognitive decline 111
　and heart health 42, 87
　menopause 45, 47, 48, 83
　and mental health 144
　and muscles 86
Okinawa, Japan 20, 22–3, 103
omega-3 fatty acids 100, 106, 110, 127
one-mile walk test 205–7, 208
osteopenia 27–8
osteoporosis 9, 32, 34, 42, 45, 47, 84
overhead presses 280–2
oxidative stress 71, 109, 110
oxytocin 146, 151, 154, 172

parents, caring for 55–6
peppers: spinach, feta & roasted pepper frittata 300–1
perimenopause 45, 46–7, 49, 83, 111
Pes, Dr Gianni 21
pesto: creamy pesto salmon with lentils & greens 307–8
　pesto salmon & roasted veg tray bake 308–9
Pilates 67, 75, 78

piriformis stretch 261–2
plank taps 283–4
plant-based diet 101, 114, 116, 117–18, 292
polyphenols 101, 110, 114
postcode lottery, life expectancy 18
posterior chain 188, 221, 254
postmenopause 45, 47–8
posture 186, 218
Poulain, Dr Michel 21
prebiotics 114, 117
pregnancy 32
press-ups 186, 200–3, 208, 269–70
probiotics 117
progesterone 46, 50, 83, 144–5
prompt-based journalling 166–7
proprioception 190, 255
protein 97, 100, 106
protein balls 312
protein-packed yoghurt bowl 296–7
puberty 45, 143
public health policies 18
pulling motion 188
push presses 287
pushing motion 187
quinoa: chickpea & quinoa chilli 302–3

reach test 198–200, 208
reflective journalling 162
relationships 55–61, 140, 153 7
resistance training 6, 28, 67, 72–4
rest and recovery 151, 175–8

reverse flys 286
reverse lunges 275–6
reverse lunges biceps 276
Romanian deadlifts 273–4
rotations 188
running 77

salad, lentil & goat's cheese 306
salmon: creamy pesto salmon with lentils & greens 307–8
    pesto salmon & roasted veg tray bake 308–9
sarcopenia 86–7
Sardinia, Italy 20, 21, 22, 103, 133
screening 35–44
sedentary lifestyle 230
sensory rest 177
serotonin 89, 115, 144, 150, 181
Seventh-Day Adventists 24, 103
shopping lists 315–16
side lunges 278–9
single-arm overhead presses 281–2
single leg stand test 190–3, 208, 231
single-leg thrusts 280
single parents 58
sit-to-stand test 193–5, 208
skin cancer 44
sleep 89, 91, 134, 141, 161, 179–82
SMART goals 318–21
smear tests 37, 38–9
smoked mackerel & sweet potato fishcakes 311–12

snacks 98, 106, 312–13
social connections 20, 22, 140, 146, 153–7
social rest 177
solo parents 58
soup, hearty vegetable 305
spinach: creamy pesto salmon with lentils & greens 307–8
spinach, feta & roasted pepper frittata 300–1
spinning 76
split squats 277–8
SPS (Serrated Polyposis Syndrome) 36
squat jumps 267
squat test 203–5, 208
squat thrusters 268–9
squats 185, 187, 230, 265–9, 277–8
stability exercises 265–90
step-parenting 59–60
stream of consciousness journalling 164–5
strength training 70, 72–4, 81, 137
  and bone health 85
  and mental health 150
  and mitochondria 90
  and muscle health 87
  and myokines 91
  strength and stability exercises 265–90
  weight training 76, 185, 213, 219–20, 231
stress 70, 89, 91, 151
stress hormones 96, 105–6, 145, 153, 171–2

stretches 86
  cooling down 222–3
  mobility and balance 253–65
  warming up 221
stroke 43, 44, 70
suitcase carry 290
sumo squats 267–8
supplements 125–7
sweet potatoes: lentil & sweet potato burrito mix 309–10
  lentil & sweet potato curry 301–2
  smoked mackerel & sweet potato fishcakes 311–12

testosterone 50, 86, 146
thoracic rotation 222, 264–5
thread the needle 221, 257–8
timed up and go (TUG) test 195–7, 208
tiredness 89
tofu: broccoli, shiitake & tofu frittata 299–300
  chickpea & tofu omelette muffins 297–8
  tofu & veggie stir-fry 304
trainers 214
trans people, breast screening 39–40
tryptophan 180
twists 188, 285–6

ultra-processed foods (UPFs) 101, 107, 129–32, 180
upright rows 271–2
US Food and Drug Administration (FDA) 32

vegetables 314–16
    hearty vegetable soup 305
    pesto salmon & roasted veg tray bake 308–9
    tofu & veggie stir-fry 304
    veggie lentil bolognese 310–11
visual journalling 168–9
vitamin A 98
vitamin B complex 99, 110, 126
vitamin C 126
vitamin D 84, 85, 98, 99, 110, 127
vitamin E 98
vitamin K 98

wake-up ritual 235
walking 67, 72, 77
    after meals 230
    gait 188
    and inflammation 90
    and joint health 86
    one-mile walk test 205–7, 208

walkouts 221, 258
warm-ups 209–10, 220–1, 234, 235
water, drinking 100, 112, 214
weight: alcohol and 135
    intermittent fasting 122
    weight-loss injections 136–7
weight training 76, 185, 213, 219–20, 231
wine 133–4, 181, 293
Women's Health Initiative (WHI) 84
World Health Organization 102, 134
world's greatest stretch 256–7

yoga 67, 75, 79, 90
yoghurt bowl, protein-packed 296–7

zinc 110

ACKNOWLEDGEMENTS

Never in a million years did I think I'd write a book, let alone two.

Whilst *Owning Your Menopause: Fitter, Calmer, Stronger* underpins everything I do, this second book truly cements what I believe we should all be working towards: a brighter, healthier future for ourselves and the generations around us.

To include my mum in this one fills my heart. Knowing it could help her stay strong and independent kept me tied to my desk, often missing other opportunities so that I could finish this. Mum, I love you so much. As my only remaining parent, I hope you continue to listen and take what I've written here to heart, because I want you to live well for as long as possible, in good health and with complete independence.

To my three incredible children, Ollie, Sophie and Rupert, thank you for putting up with me talking (and on!) about longevity, muscle strength and gut health. I know there were moments you were snorting at me, but I hope, deep down, you've taken it all in. You are the reason I want this message to be heard. In my world, you will live long, pain-free and disease-free lives.

To my husband, hopefully you now *fully* understand the importance of weights! Your support always means the world. And yes, I'm sorry for the bad morning music choices . . . but I do need them.

To my sister, I just love you. Even though you're far away, I know you're always there, helping in quiet ways no one else sees. For that, I am eternally grateful. You are the yin to my yang, the calm to my storm.

Daddy, you never learned about book one... and now here I am with book two. I know you'd be so proud. You were on my mind often while writing this, especially the parts about tuning in, paying attention and questioning anything that doesn't feel right. That's what you always taught me.

To Nicky Way, my brilliant book agent, your patience, belief and friendship have meant everything. I didn't always think I had this, but you never stopped believing. I can't wait to see what we create next.

To Nicky Ross, thank you for seeing the potential in this idea and helping me bring it to life. You trusted me to deliver another much-needed book, and I have high hopes for what it can do.

To all at Becca Barr Management, thank you for keeping me supported and grounded, especially during those waves of impostor syndrome. Your advice has been so valuable, and I am grateful for your belief in me.

Finally, to my amazing *Owning Your Menopause* community, thank you for continuing to show me that what I do makes a difference. You are living proof that change is possible and that women around the world are ready to take back their power.

ABOUT THE AUTHOR

Kate Rowe-Ham is a leading Women's Health Coach, menopause fitness specialist and bestselling author of *Owning Your Menopause: Fitter, Calmer, Stronger in 30 Days*. She is also the founder of the *Owning Your Menopause* app and host of the *Owning Your Menopause* podcast, where she shares evidence-based strategies and empowering conversations that help women thrive through midlife and beyond.

Kate's journey into health coaching began with her own experience navigating perimenopause while raising three children and qualifying as a Level 3 Personal Trainer later in life. Confronted by the lack of clear, evidence-based support for women, she made it her mission to become the voice of clarity, compassion and empowerment in menopause and women's health.

At the heart of Kate's work lies a passion that extends beyond menopause, a commitment to helping women future-proof their bodies and minds for lifelong vitality and well-being. She teaches women in a positive and doable way how to build the foundations for strength, independence and resilience by focusing on what truly matters: movement for mobility and longevity, food that fuels hormonal balance, and mindset practices that promote calm, confidence and clarity.

A trusted and respected voice in women's health, Kate is regularly featured across leading national and international media, including *The Times*, *The Telegraph*, *The Daily Mail*,

HELLO!, Women's Health, Good Housekeeping, Prima, Woman & Home, Women's Fitness, Liz Earle Wellbeing, Fit & Well and Coach. She is part of the Women's Health magazine collective, writes a monthly column as one of Top Santé's 'Three Wise Women' and serves as a proud Patron of Menopause Mandate, championing better awareness, education and support for women nationwide.

Kate's expertise and relatable approach have earned her collaborations with global brands including Nike, Sweaty Betty, Lucozade Sport, FatFace, JD Williams, and wellness pioneers such as Ancient + Brave. Her media presence spans BBC News, ITV, Channel 4's Sunday Brunch, Katie Piper's Weekend Retreat, BBC Radio, and LBC Radio, as well as features in The Times, The Telegraph, Women's Health, Fit & Well, Prima, Good Housekeeping, Woman & Home, Liz Earle Wellbeing and Coach. She has also appeared on podcasts, including The Mid Point with Gaby Logan, RunPod with Jenni Falconer, Sober Dave, Wild Nutrition and Lawrence Price.

As a sought-after speaker, Kate regularly inspires audiences at leading health and wellness events, including CarFest, Ideas Fest, Postcards from Midlife, The Big Retreat Festival, and The Joe Wicks Festival. Her expertise has also attracted a high profile client base, including actress Tamzin Outhwaite and TV presenter Laura Hamilton.

Kate's mission is clear: to redefine how women experience menopause, transforming it from a time of decline into an opportunity to flourish. Through education, empowerment and sustainable lifestyle strategies, she helps women unlock their potential to be strong in both body and mind at every stage of life.

Instagram: @katerh_fitness
Website: www.owningyourmenopause.com

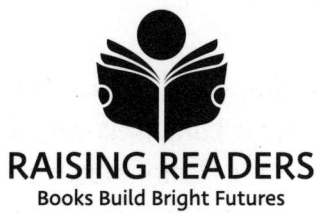

RAISING READERS
Books Build Bright Futures

Dear Reader,

We'd love your attention for one more page to tell you about the crisis in children's reading, and what we can all do.

Studies have shown that reading for fun is the **single biggest predictor of a child's future life chances** – more than family circumstance, parents' educational background or income. It improves academic results, mental health, wealth, communication skills, ambition and happiness.[1]

The number of children reading for fun is in rapid decline. Young people have a lot of competition for their time. In 2024, 1 in 10 children and young people in the UK aged 5 to 18 did not own a single book at home.[2]

Hachette works extensively with schools, libraries and literacy charities, but here are some ways we can all raise more readers:

- Reading to children for just 10 minutes a day makes a difference
- Don't give up if children aren't regular readers – there will be books for them!
- Visit bookshops and libraries to get recommendations
- Encourage them to listen to audiobooks
- Support school libraries
- Give books as gifts

There's a lot more information about how to encourage children to read on our website: **www.RaisingReaders.co.uk**

Thank you for reading.

hachette UK

---

[1] OECD, '21st-Century Readers: Developing Literacy Skills in a Digital World', 2021, https://www.oecd.org/en/publications/21st-century-readers_a83d84cb-en.html

[2] National Literacy Trust, 'Book Ownership in 2024', November 2024, https://literacytrust.org.uk/research-services/research-reports/book-ownership-in-2024